Bones and Joints

A Guide for Students

SIXTH EDITION

Chris Gunn MA TDCR

Formerly CGTraining, Nottinghamshire, UK

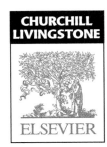

CHURCHILL
LIVINGSTONE

ELSEVIER

EDINBURGH LONDON NEW YORK OXFORD PHILADELPHIA
ST LOUIS SYDNEY TORONTO 2012

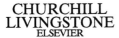

First edition 1984
Second edition 1992
Third edition 1996
Fourth edition 2002
Fifth edition 2007
Sixth edition 2012
Reprinted 2014, 2015

ISBN 978 0 7020 4311 6

British Library Cataloguing in Publication Data
A catalogue record for this book is available from the British Library

Library of Congress Cataloging in Publication Data
A catalog record for this book is available from the Library of Congress

Notices
Knowledge and best practice in this field are constantly changing. As new research and experience broaden our understanding, changes in research methods, professional practices, or medical treatment may become necessary.

Practitioners and researchers must always rely on their own experience and knowledge in evaluating and using any information, methods, compounds, or experiments described herein. In using such information or methods they should be mindful of their own safety and the safety of others, including parties for whom they have a professional responsibility.

With respect to any drug or pharmaceutical products identified, readers are advised to check the most current information provided (i) on procedures featured or (ii) by the manufacturer of each product to be administered, to verify the recommended dose or formula, the method and duration of administration, and contraindications. It is the responsibility of practitioners, relying on their own experience and knowledge of their patients, to make diagnoses, to determine dosages and the best treatment for each individual patient, and to take all appropriate safety precautions.

To the fullest extent of the law, neither the Publisher nor the authors, contributors, or editors, assume any liability for any injury and/or damage to persons or property as a matter of products liability, negligence or otherwise, or from any use or operation of any methods, products, instructions, or ideas contained in the material herein.

 your source for books, journals and multimedia in the health sciences

www.elsevierhealth.com

Working together to grow
libraries in developing countries

www.elsevier.com | www.bookaid.org | www.sabre.org

ELSEVIER   BOOK AID International   Sabre Foundation

The Publisher's policy is to use paper manufactured from sustainable forests

Printed in Great Britain

Bones and Joints

For Elsevier

Commissioning Editor: Claire Wilson
Development Editor: Fiona Conn
Project Manager: Nancy Arnott
Designer: Charles Gray
Illustration Manager: Merlyn Harvey
Illustrator: Robert Britton

Preface

The aim of this book has always been to demystify the topic of bones and joints. In this edition I am pleased to be able to include some examples of PET and SPECT images, some replacement radiographs and pathology, and improve the quality of the line drawings. When selecting the illustrations I have had to bear in mind that this is essentially a book about bones and joints and it is not a pathology text. I have therefore tried to select examples showing obvious pathology and utilising different imaging techniques. It must be stressed that early signs of pathology often present in a much more subtle way and I would encourage readers to look at the radiographs alongside the pathology sections.

I have always felt that osteology and arthrology can be best studied by using a systematic and logical approach to the subject and by handling the individual bones. I have attempted to provide a logical framework and it is hoped that those using the book will have access to samples of individual bones.

All the major bones and joints of the human body have been covered including a section on teeth. The text has been written in note form and the diagrams have been made as clear and simple as possible so that they can be easily reproduced by students.

The book can be used in several ways depending on the individual:

1. As part of a self-learning programme in conjunction with actual bones and supported by follow-up tutorials.
2. As part of a revision programme on completion of a course of study (the legends on the diagrams have been lettered, with the actual terminology listed at the side of the drawing to allow self-testing).
3. As a reference book.

I would like to thank Philips Healthcare for Plates 1, 4, 6, 7, and 8; Philip Panto for his support and very constructive comments on the text and for providing Figures 3.8, 3.26, 4.14; Carl Miller for providing the radiographs for Figure 3.1, 3.8, 3.18, 3.22, 3.26, 4.9, 4.31, 4.33, 5.3, 5.11, 6.15, 6.16, 6.19 and 6.20; Vidhiya Vinayakamoorthy and InHealth for Plates 2, 3 and 5; Glenda Bryan for permission to use radiographs from Bryan GJ 1996, Skeletal Anatomy for Figures 1.6, 4.3, 4.4, 4.7, 4.8, 4.12, 4.13, 4.18, 4.19, 4.20, 4.21, 4.25, 4.26, 4.27, 4.28, 4.29, 5.4, 5.7, 5.8, 5.12, 5.13, 5.18, 5.20, 6.3, 6.4, 6.5, 6.6, 6.11, 6.12, 6.21, 6.22, 6.30, 6.31, 6.32, 6.33, 6.37, 6.40, 6.41, 6.42, 7.6, 7.7, 7.12, 7.13, 7.14, 7.18, 7.19, 7.20, 8.3, 8.4, 8.8, 8.9, 8.10, 9.3, 9.4, 9.5, 9.6, 9.10, 9.11, 9.15, 9.16, 9.17, 9.20, 9.21, 9.22, 9.23, 9.26, 9.27, 9.28, 9.31, 9.34, 10.5, 10.6, 10.10, 10.11, 10.12, 10.13, 10.14,

10.15, 10.16, 10.17, 10.18, 10.24, 10.25, 10.26, 10.27, 10.29, 10.30, 10.36, 10.37, 10.38, 10.46, 10.49, 10.50, 10.51, 10.52, 10.53, 10.55, 10.56; Ernest Higginbottom for providing the radiographs for Figures 1.4, 1.5, 3.7, 3.10, 3.15, 3.16, 3.19, 3.23, 3.28, 6.24, 6.25, 7.15, 7.17, 9.40, 9.41, 9.42, 9.44; Agfa Gevaert for assisting with the production of the final prints from those radiographs; Elsevier and the original contributors for permission to use the illustrations from Sutton (ed) 1987 A Textbook of Radiology and Imaging for Figures 3.3, 3.5, 3.9, 3.12, 3.17, 3.20, 3.21, 3.24, 3.25, 4.10, 4.32, 4.35, 6.44 and 10.59 and from Resnick, Kransdorf 2005 Bone and Joint Imaging for Figures 3.2, 3.4, 3.6, 3.11, 3.13, 3.14, 3.27, 4.22, 4.30, 4.34, 5.14, 5.15, 5.16, 5.21, 6.7, 6.8, 6.17, 6.23, 6.34, 6.35, 6.36, 6.43, 6.45, 7.16, 7.21, 9.12, 9.29, 9.35, 9.36, 9.37, 9.38, 9.39, 9.43, 9.45, 10.57, 10.58 and 10.60. I would also like to thank those colleagues who assisted with the first edition of Bones and Joints: M G McKenzie, Mr M Mathews, Miss M Ledger and Mr J Young; and finally my thanks to Dr D A Gunn who drew the original diagrams.

Chris Gunn
Nottinghamshire 2011

Contents

Bone

CHAPTER CONTENTS

Bone is a highly vascular connective tissue, in which bone cells are enclosed in a mineralised intercellular matrix interposed with a system of collagenous fibres.

The organic matrix forms one-third of the structure and gives resilience and a degree of flexibility; the mineral salts (mainly calcium and phosphorus) form the remaining two-thirds and provide the strength and weightbearing capabilities of the bone.

STRUCTURE OF BONE

There are two main types of bone: *compact* (dense) and *cancellous* (spongy). Compact bone forms the surface layers or cortex of mature bones and cancellous bone the interior aspect.

Compact bone

This type of bone is found mainly in the shafts of long bones where a strong, tubular structure is required. It consists of a number of cylindrical structures called *haversian systems* (Figs 1.1 and 1.2). Each system comprises:

A central haversian canal –
which contains blood, lymphatic vessels and nerves.

Lamellae –
rings of bone round the haversian canal.

Lacunae –
spaces between the lamellae, which contain osteocytes (mature bone cells).

Canaliculi –
channels carrying nutrient fluid, which connect the lacunae and communicate with the haversian canal.

Interstitial lamellae –
fill the spaces between adjacent *haversian systems.*

Circumferential lamellae –
rings of bone round the edge of the bone.

Volkmann's canals –
join the various haversian canals.

Periosteum –

a membrane which surrounds the bone, except at the articular surfaces, where articular hyaline cartilage allows friction-free movement. The inner layer is vascular and cellular providing nutrition, growth and repair. The outer layer is fibrous and blends with tendons and ligaments.

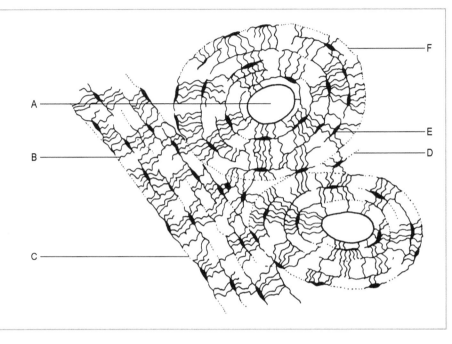

Fig. 1.1 Transverse section of bone (microscopic).
A – Haversian canal
B – Canaliculi
C – Circumferential lamella
D – Interstitial lamella
E – Lacuna
F – Lamella.

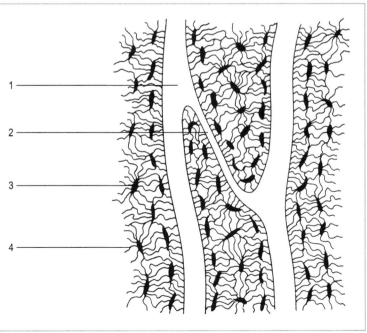

Fig. 1.2 Longitudinal section of bone (microscopic).
1 – Haversian canal
2 – Volkmann's canal
3 – Lacuna
4 – Canaliculi.

Cancellous bone

This type of bone is found in the parts of bones where lightness, strength and area are required. It is similar in structure to compact bone but bone marrow is found between the trabeculae which form the internal support structure of the bone.

Bone marrow

The medullary cavity of bone and the spaces between the trabeculae of cancellous bone are filled with bone marrow. At birth this is red bone marrow, which produces red and white blood cells.

In adults, active red bone marrow is found only in the:

- upper femora
- vertebrae
- scapulae
- sternum
- ribs
- clavicles
- diploë of skull bones
- hip bones.

Elsewhere the red bone marrow becomes inactive yellow marrow.

Development

Some bones develop from rods of cartilage, e.g. the bones which form the limbs, the trunk and the base of the skull. Some bones develop from membranes, e.g. bones of the vault of the skull, the face and the clavicle. Some bones develop in tendons, e.g. sesamoid bones – the patella and fabella.

Ossification

Ossification is the formation of bone from connective tissue and requires:

- adequate calcium and phosphate in the blood
- a supply of vitamins A, C and D.

Growth of the bone is influenced by the following hormones:

Parathormone (from the parathyroid glands) – controls the level of calcium, and indirectly the level of phosphates in the blood.

Growth hormone (from the anterior lobe of the pituitary gland) – influences growth and replacement of bone tissue.

Thyroxine (from the thyroid gland) – influences normal physical development.

Testosterone (in the male) and oestrogen (in the female) – influences normal skeletal growth especially at puberty.

Weightbearing and exercise also stimulate bone growth and general ill health inhibits it.

Intramembranous ossification

This takes place in a membrane, e.g. in the vault of the skull in the developing fetus. At the point of ossification, osteogenic fibres and bone cells appear in the connective tissue and calcium salts are deposited to form osteoid tissue. Ossification spreads from the centre outwards.

Intracartilaginous ossification

The process by which bone formation takes place, e.g. in a long bone (Fig. 1.3).

Primary centre of ossification

This appears in the middle of the *diaphysis*. Osteoblasts (bone cells) appear and calcium is laid down.

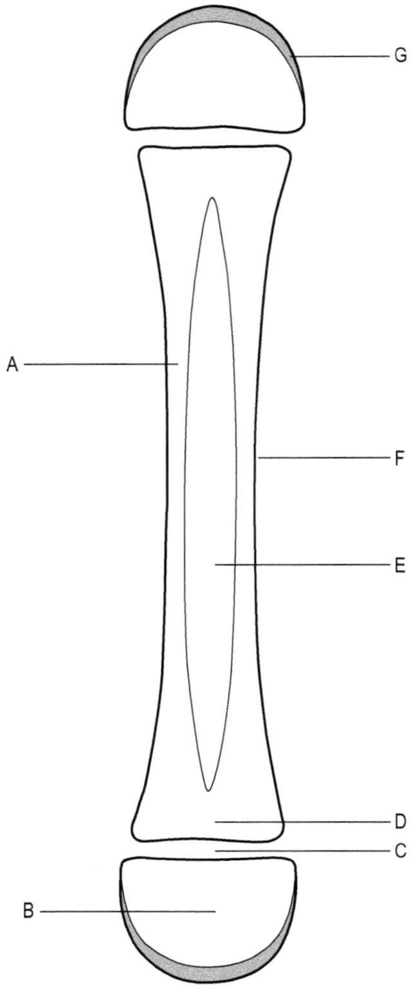

Fig. 1.3 Section through a developing long bone.
A – Diaphysis
B – Epiphysis
C – Epiphyseal plate
D – Metaphysis
E – Medullary cavity
F – Periosteum
G – Articular hyaline cartilage.

Osteoblasts 'build the bone' by laying down fibres, matrix and calcium.

Osteoclasts are a type of cell which 'destroy the bone' and therefore mould the bone into the required shape – 'remodelling'.

Osteoclasts are responsible for forming the *medullary canals* and *sinuses* within the bone.

At the same time as the diaphysis is being formed, bone is being built up on the outside of the shaft, which later forms the *periosteum*.

Secondary centres of ossification

These appear at the ends of the bone and form the *epiphyses* (singular epiphysis). The epiphysis is separated from the diaphysis by a thin layer of cartilage called the *epiphyseal plate*.

Growth

This occurs during childhood by the production of bone at the epiphyseal plate. It occurs at the side of the epiphyseal plate nearest the shaft, which is called the *metaphysis*.

Fusion

The fusion of the epiphysis with the diaphysis occurs when the bone reaches the desired size. A typical long bone can take up to 20 years to reach fusion.

Function of bone

Bone:

- supports soft tissue
- supports the body weight
- enables movement
- protects organs, e.g. the brain
- stores calcium
- produces blood cells from the red bone marrow.

Blood supply

The blood to the bone supplies:

- bone tissue
- bone cells
- bone marrow
- epiphyseal cartilage
- periosteum.

There are several distinct points where the large blood vessels enter the bone, called the nutrient foramina. These usually point away from the dominant growing end of the bone. Numerous smaller vessels enter through the non-articular surfaces of the epiphyses.

The arterial blood feeds the bone and then drains into venous channels which leave the bone through the surfaces which are not covered with articular hyaline cartilage.

Nerve supply

Nerves are widely distributed in the periosteum and nerve fibres accompany the arteries into the bone via the nutrient foramen.

TYPES OF BONES

Long bones

These consist of a shaft of compact bone with a central medullary cavity. The expanded ends are formed by cancellous bone covered with compact bone.

Examples

humerus	fibula
radius	phalanges
ulna	metatarsals
femur	metacarpals
tibia	clavicle.

Short bones (cuboidal shape)	These are formed by cancellous bone with a thin covering of compact bone, giving strength but with limited movement. *Examples* carpal bones tarsal bones.
Flat bones	These have a thin layer of cancellous bone enclosed in two thin layers of compact bone and are found where protection for underlying organs or extensive muscle attachment is required. *Examples* scapulae ribs vault of the skull.
Irregular bones	These are composed of cancellous bone surrounded by a thin layer of compact bone. *Examples* vertebrae facial bones hip bones.
Sesamoid bones	These develop in tendons, usually near a joint, and their main function is to protect the tendon from wear as it moves over the bony surface. *Examples* patella fabella.

'NORMAL' RADIOGRAPHIC BONE APPEARANCES (Figs 1.4, 1.5 and 1.6)

Cortex – is more dense than the medullary cavity and therefore absorbs more radiation, producing a reasonably solid 'white line' round the periphery of the bone.

Medullary cavity – is less dense than the cortex and therefore appears slightly darker.

Cancellous bone – the trabeculae, which are the support structure of the cancellous bone, have the appearance of very fine 'white lines' throughout the bone.

Epiphyseal plate – as this is formed by cartilage it is radiolucent and therefore care must be taken not to confuse it with a fracture. It has the appearance of a radiolucent area with 2 fairly regular margins, extending to the periphery of the bone and situated near the ends.

Fused epiphyses – appear, usually, during the teenage years, and occur as a thin 'white line' along the site of the old epiphyseal plate. With age these lines are no longer visible.

Joint cavity – this contains articular hyaline cartilage and synovial fluid and is radiolucent (and therefore not demonstrated).

Fig. 1.4 Normal bone appearances, left foot. (Courtesy of Ernest Higginbottom.)
A – Cortex
B – Medullary cavity (cancellous bone)
C – Joint cavity.

Fig. 1.5 Normal bone appearances, ankle. (Courtesy of Ernest Higginbottom.)
A – Fused epiphysis
B – Epiphysis.

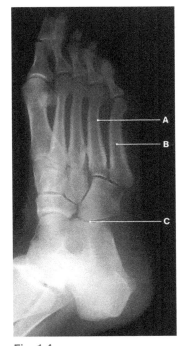

Fig. 1.4

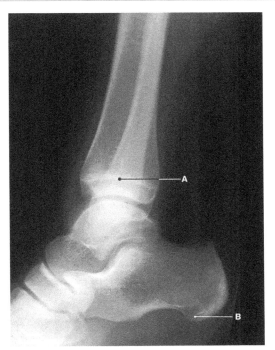

Fig. 1.5

Fig. 1.6 Radiograph of the upper end of femur. (From Bryan 1996.)
A – Compact bone
B – Spongy bone
C – Medullary cavity.

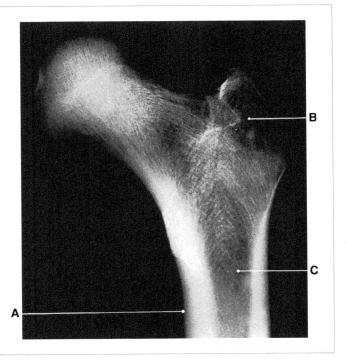

TERMINOLOGY

INSIGHT

Learning these terms will enable the reader to work out the names of different parts of a bone.

The names of most aspects of bone can be built up logically from a combination of some of the following:

- an adjective derived from the name of the bone
- an adjective derived from the bone with which they articulate
- an adjective derived from part of the bone with which they articulate
- a prefix
- a descriptive term – see lists below (elevations, projections, holes and depressions).

Examples

Subscapular fossa – a depression below the scapula

Trochlear notch – a large groove which articulates with the trochlea

Radial fossa – a depression which receives the head of radius

Supracondylar ridge – a ridge above a condyle.

Elevations and projections

Auricular – ear-shaped

Condyle – a smooth, rounded elevation, often covered with articular hyaline cartilage

Crest – a sharp ridge

Epicondyle – an elevation above a condyle

Facet – a smooth area, usually covered with articular hyaline cartilage

Hamulus – a hook-like projection

Lamina – a thin plate

Line – a low, narrow ridge

Process – a localised projection

Spine – an elongated process

Squamous – thin, flat, like a scale

Trochanter – a large rounded elevation

Trochlea – a pulley-shaped surface

Tubercle – a small rounded elevation

Tuberosity – a large rounded elevation.

Holes or depressions

Canal – a bony tunnel

Fissure – a narrow slit

Foramen – a hole

Fossa – a wide depression

Groove – an uncovered passage

Meatus – a narrow passage

Notch – a large groove

Sulcus – a groove or furrow.

Prefixes

Demi – half

Epi – above

Infra – below

Inter – between

Intra – within

Sub – below

Supra – above.

Descriptive terms

Anterior – nearer the front of the body

Costal – associated with the ribs

Distal – away from the trunk

Dorsal – nearer the back of the body

External – outside

Inferior – below

Internal – inside

Lateral – away from the midline of the body

Medial – nearer the midline of the body

Posterior – nearer the back of the body

Proximal – towards the trunk

Superior – above

Ventral – nearer the front of the body.

Terms associated with teeth

Buccal/labial – adjacent to the lips or cheeks

Cusps – rounded projections

Distal – towards the back of the mouth

Lingual/palatal – next to the tongue

Mesial – towards the front or the midline

Occlusal – biting edge.

Joints

CHAPTER CONTENTS

A joint is formed where two or more bones meet and is classified as being synovial, fibrous or cartilaginous in nature.

The main types of joints found in the body are classified as synovial joints.

SYNOVIAL JOINTS (DIARTHROSES)

Features of a typical synovial joint (Fig. 2.1)

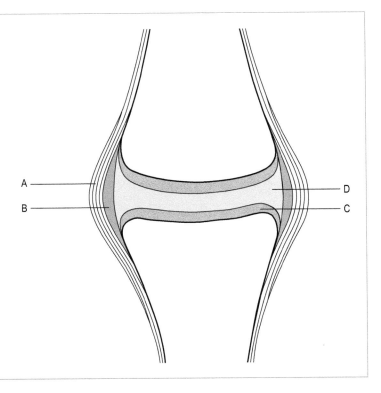

Fig. 2.1 **Typical synovial joint (coronal section).**
A – Fibrous capsule
B – Synovial membrane
C – Articular hyaline cartilage
D – Synovial fluid.

Articular hyaline cartilage covers the articular surfaces.

A fibrous capsule surrounds the joint.

Synovial membrane lines the joint, except where articular hyaline cartilage is found.

A lubricant film of synovial fluid is secreted into the joint cavity by the synovial membrane.

Ligaments strengthen the joint capsule. These may be separate from the capsule or may blend with it.

Movement occurs at the joint but the amount varies with the type of synovial joint.

Nerves and blood vessels supply the joint.

Intracapsular structures may be present, e.g. tendons, ligaments, joint discs, pads of fat.

Movements of the joints

Flexion – bending the joint, i.e. decreasing the angle between the bones.

Extension – straightening the joint, i.e. increasing the angle between the bones.

Abduction – to move away from the midline.

Adduction – to move towards the midline.

Internal rotation – to turn inwards.

External rotation – to turn outwards.

Circumduction – a combination of the above movements.

Gliding – one articular surface sliding smoothly over another.

Types of synovial joints

Synovial hinge joints

Uniaxial joints (movement round one axis).

Movements –
flexion and extension.

Examples
elbow joint
interphalangeal joints.

Synovial condylar joints

Uniaxial joints.

Movements –
flexion, extension and rotation.

Examples
knee joint
temporomandibular joint.

Synovial ellipsoid joints

Biaxial joints (movement round 2 axes).

Movements –
flexion, extension, abduction and adduction.

Examples
wrist joint
metacarpophalangeal joints
metatarsophalangeal joints
atlanto-occipital joint.

Synovial saddle joints

Biaxial joints

Movements –
flexion, extension, abduction, adduction and a degree of axial rotation.

Examples
1st carpometacarpal joint
calcaneocuboid joint
sternoclavicular joint
ankle joint.

Synovial pivot joints

Uniaxial joints

Movements –
rotation only.

Examples
superior radio-ulnar joint
inferior radio-ulnar joint
median atlanto-axial joint (the odontoid process on the arch of the atlas).

Synovial ball and socket joints

Multiaxial joints (movement around more than 2 axes).

Movements –
flexion, extension, abduction, adduction, rotation and circumduction.

Examples
hip joint
shoulder joint.

Synovial plane joints

Movements –
gliding only.

Examples
sacroiliac joint
superior tibiofibular joint

cubonavicular joint
tarsometatarsal joints
acromioclavicular joints
2nd–5th carpometacarpal joints
joints between the vertebral arches (lateral atlanto-axial joints)
costovertebral joints.

FIBROUS JOINTS (SYNARTHROSES)

These joints usually have virtually no movement. The bones are joined by fibrous tissue.

Types of fibrous joints

Sutures

Movements –
limited movement up to about the age of 20, then the joints become fixed.
Examples
limited to joints between bones of the skull.

Gomphoses

Movements –
minimal.
Examples
between the teeth and the jaws.

Syndesmoses

In these joints the bones are held together by an interosseous ligament or membrane.
Movements –
variable.
Examples
inferior tibiofibular joint
middle tibiofibular and radio-ulnar joints.

CARTILAGINOUS JOINTS (AMPHIARTHROSES)

These joints either have no movement or minimal movement and are joined by a layer of cartilage.

Types of cartilaginous joints

Synchondrosis

Movements –
absent or minimal.
Examples
sternocostal joints (minimal movement)
joint between the diaphysis and epiphysis of a growing long bone – a temporary joint with *no* movement.

Symphysis

The ends of the bone are covered with articular hyaline cartilage and are joined by a disc of fibrocartilage and surrounding ligaments.

Movements –
variable.

Examples
joints between the vertebral bodies
sacrococcygeal joint
symphysis pubis
manubriosternal joint.

Pathology

CHAPTER CONTENTS

Pathology is the study of disease. This chapter covers some of the more common diseases which can be detected radiographically. Pathology concerning specific areas of the body will be discussed in later chapters following the relevant bone or joint. Radiographs have been included to demonstrate some of the pathology; these are often advanced examples and it should be remembered that early signs will not be as obvious.

CHANGES DUE TO PATHOLOGY

Loss of bone density

This is usually a decrease in the amount of calcium present in the bone and therefore the bone becomes less dense in structure. The bone is more radiolucent and therefore appears 'darker' on a radiograph. This may be an overall loss of density or be specific to particular areas of bone.

Osteoporosis
(Figs 3.1, 3.2)

A deficiency in the bone matrix due to a reduction in bone formation – therefore the bones fracture easily.

Causes – lack of vitamin C (scurvy). Old age. Disuse, for example due to immobilisation following fracture; if activity returns the bone returns to normal. Cushing's syndrome. Overuse of steroid hormones. Post-menopausal, related to reduced oestrogen levels.

Radiological signs – bone affected appears radiolucent. The primary trabeculae may appear more prominent.

Fig. 3.1 **Osteoporosis, resulting in a compression fracture of the first lumbar vertebra.**

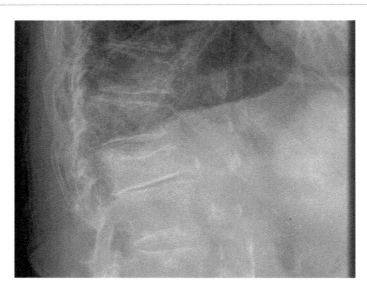

Fig. 3.2 **Osteoporosis, femoral head.** MR image. Note the joint effusion. (From Resnick Kransdorf, 2005.)

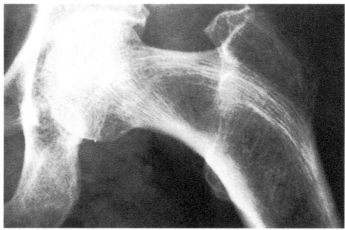

Osteomalacia ('adult rickets') (Fig. 3.3)

An overall decrease in bone calcification.

Causes – diet low in vitamin D, calcium or phosphorus. Malabsorption syndromes, e.g. coeliac disease, Crohn's disease, renal disease.

Radiological signs – narrow bands of decalcification 2–3 mm wide called Looser's zones ('pseudo fractures').

Osteogenesis imperfecta (Fig. 3.4)

Bone formation is defective. The bones become small, thin and prone to fracture. Growth becomes stunted and limb deformity results.

Cause – congenital disorders (rare).

Fig. 3.3 Osteomalacia, ulnar shaft.
(From Sutton 1987.)

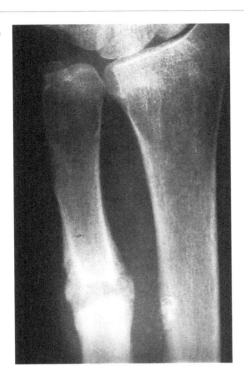

Fig. 3.4 Osteogenesis imperfecta, lower extremities. Note a decrease in bone density associated with thin long bones, multiple fractures and bowing of the long bones. (From Resnick Kransdorf, 2005.)

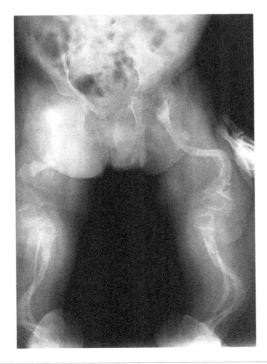

Osteitis fibrosa cystica

Loss of bone density due to the increase in blood calcium, the bones becoming decalcified. The skull appears mottled; bones develop cystic areas; bone is reabsorbed. Pathological fractures may occur.

Cause – hyperparathyroidism: overactivity of the parathyroid glands and therefore excessive secretion of parathormone.

Increase in bone density

This is usually an increase in the amount of calcium present in the bone (osteosclerosis), resulting in the bone becoming denser in structure. The bone becomes more radiopaque and therefore appears 'whiter' on the radiograph.

Osteopetrosis (Fig. 3.5)

Increased density of bones which have been ossified from cartilage, but mainly in the ribs, pelvis, and vertebrae. Bones become hard but brittle and therefore fracture easily. A prominent line of calcification can often be seen along the epiphyseal plate.

Cause – disturbances when the bones are being formed during pregnancy.

Radiological signs – appearance of 'bone within a bone'.

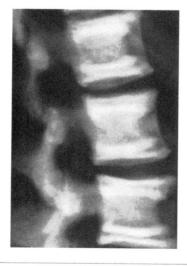

Fig. 3.5 Osteopetrosis, vertebral bodies.
(From Sutton 1987.)

Fluorosis

A generalised increase in bone density. Mottled discolouration of the teeth occurs.

Cause – excessive ingestion of fluorine.

Lead poisoning (Fig. 3.6)

Radiographically dense transverse lines appear at the ends of the shafts of long bones.

Cause – excessive lead intake.

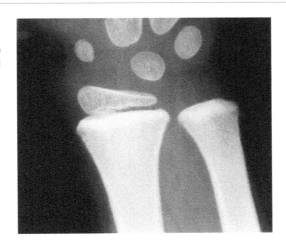

Fig. 3.6 Lead poisoning, wrist. Note dense transverse lines on the radius and ulna. (From Resnick Kransdorf, 2005.)

Myelosclerosis	*A generalised increase in bone density. Secondary bone sclerosis and anaemia occur.*
Paget's disease (Figs 3.7, 3.8)	Sometimes described as a 'cotton wool' skull; some absorption of bone and excessive deposition of new bone occurs. There is increased vascularity and therefore increased bone destruction followed by bone repair with abnormal bone pattern and coarse, thickened trabeculae. It usually affects the skull, femora, tibiae, lumbar spine and pelvis and is common in old age.

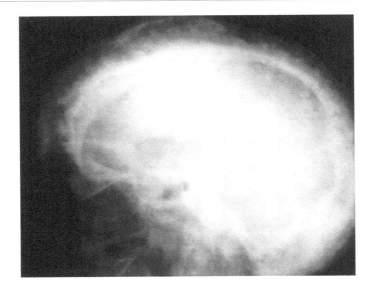

Fig. 3.7 Paget's disease, skull. (Courtesy of Ernest Higginbottom.)

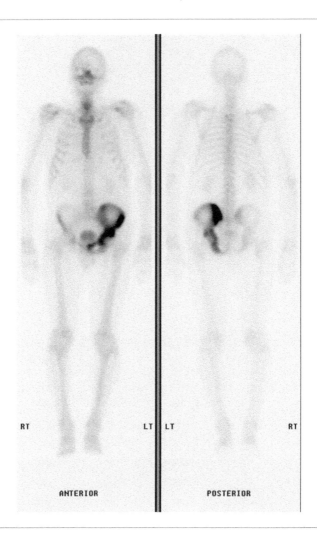

Fig. 3.8 **Paget's disease.** Skeletal scintigraphy. Note increased uptake of radionuclide throughout the left hemi-pelvis.

RT | LT | LT | RT

ANTERIOR | POSTERIOR

Bone destruction

Necrosis of the femoral head following fracture

'Bone death' due to a poor blood supply. Radiographically the bone surfaces appear irregular.

Bone tuberculosis (Fig. 3.9)

Irregular bone destruction with little new bone formation. Most common sites are the vertebral bodies, long bones, fingers and joints.

Cause – spread via the bloodstream from a tuberculous focus, usually in the lungs.

Radiological signs – if the cartilage is destroyed the bones appear to be crowded.

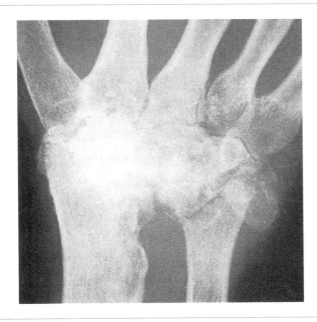

Fig. 3.9 Bone tuberculosis, wrist and carpal bones.
(From Sutton 1987.)

Osteomyelitis
(Figs 3.10, 3.11, Plate 1)

Bone infection, most common in children, usually from a Staphylococcus infection. It begins in the medullary cavity and may spread to the cortex and the periosteum. Bone destruction appears after 7 days when the periosteum becomes elevated. It can be treated with antibiotics and therefore gross bone destruction is now rare.

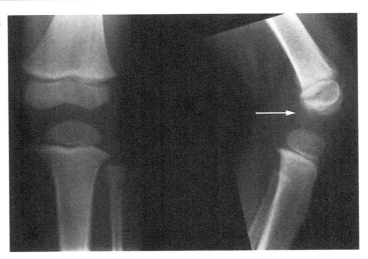

Fig. 3.10 Osteomyelitis, infant knee.
(Courtesy of Ernest Higginbottom.)

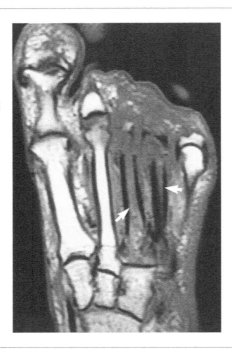

Fig. 3.11 **Recurrent diabetic bone infection following amputation of the third toe at the level of the metatarsophalangeal joint, third and fourth metatarsal and head of second metatarsal.** MR image. (From Resnick Kransdorf, 2005.)

Caisson disease (bone necrosis) (Fig. 3.12)

Affects workers who experience high atmospheric pressure, e.g. divers and tunnel workers. Radiological signs appear late and include fatigue fractures, irregular areas of callus, necrosis with adjacent fibrous collapse and degenerative changes.

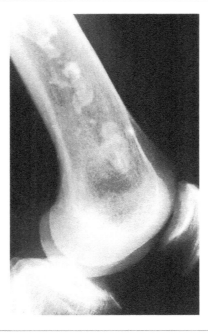

Fig. 3.12 **Caisson disease, femur.** (From Sutton 1987.)

HORMONE DISTURBANCES

Pituitary gland

The anterior lobe of the pituitary gland produces the growth hormone, which controls the rate of growth of the epiphyseal cartilage.

Gigantism

This occurs if hypersecretion takes place during childhood resulting in excessive growth.

Acromegaly
(Fig. 3.13)

This occurs if hypersecretion takes place during adulthood. It results in enlarged and thickened bones, especially the hands and mandible, and dorsal kyphosis. Enlargement of the pituitary fossa occurs because the hypersecretion is caused by an adenoma (benign tumour).

Dwarfism
(Fig. 3.14)

This occurs if hyposecretion takes place during childhood, resulting in a lack of bone growth and therefore a small individual.

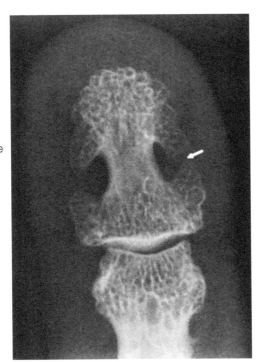

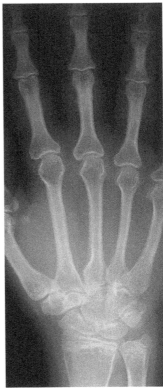

Fig. 3.13 Acromegaly, distal phalanx, hand. Note prominence of the soft tissue, enlargement of the base of the phalanx, pseudoforamina, arrowed. (From Resnick Kransdorf, 2005.)

Fig. 3.14 Hypopituitarism, wrist. Note the absence of closure of the epiphyses of the radius and ulna in a 23-year old-woman. (From Resnick Kransdorf, 2005.)

Fig. 3.13

Fig. 3.14

Thyroid gland

Cretinism   Thyroxine from the thyroid gland is responsible for normal skeletal development and therefore hyposecretion results in retarded skeletal development.

Parathyroid glands

Hyperparathyroidism   Parathormone regulates the quantity of calcium and phosphorus in the blood and bones. Hypersecretion results in a calcium loss from bones causing a radio-lucent appearance, subperiosteal bone reabsorption, deformity and fractures.

Adrenal glands

Osteoporosis   Prolonged hypersecretion of glucocorticosteroids affects calcium metabolism (as can large doses of steroids) resulting in osteoporosis of the axial skeleton.

VITAMIN DEFICIENCIES

Vitamins C and D are responsible for the formation of healthy bone tissue.

Vitamin D deficiency   Vitamin D is found in, for example, milk, eggs, fish, liver, oil and is produced by the body when the skin is exposed to ultraviolet rays from the sun. A decrease in the vitamin can result in osteomalacia (in adults), a loss of bone density or rickets (in children), when the epiphyses become enlarged and the legs bow.
Radiological signs – poorly calcified metaphysis and increase in size of the epiphyseal plate.

Vitamin C deficiency   Vitamin C is found in, for example, fresh fruit and vegetables. A decrease may result in scurvy.
Radiological signs – the periosteum is raised and osteoporosis is present.

JOINT DISORDERS

Septic arthritis   Inflammation of a joint due to a bacterial infection.

Osteoarthritis (Fig. 3.15)   Degeneration of the articular hyaline cartilage. The bone becomes thickened and spreads outwards forming 'spurs' round the joint margins. Synovial fluid may enter the bone giving it a cystic appearance. It is more common above the age of 60; the most common sites are the hips, knees and spine.

Rheumatoid arthritis (Fig. 3.16)   Radiographically, this has the appearance of bone erosion, joint deformity and a narrowed joint space due to inflammatory tissue forming over and destroying the articular hyaline cartilage and eventually replacing it, causing the joint to swell and limiting its degree of movement. It affects several joints at once. The most common sites are the fingers, ankles, hips and knees.

Fig. 3.15 Osteo-arthritis, pelvis and hips.
(Courtesy of Ernest Higginbottom.)

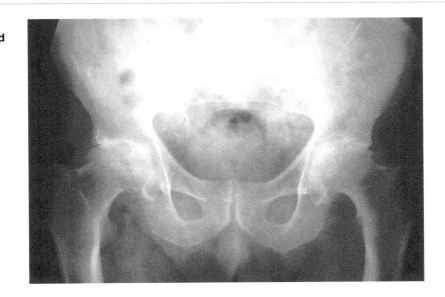

Fig. 3.16 Rheumatoid arthritis, hands.
(Courtesy of Ernest Higginbottom.)

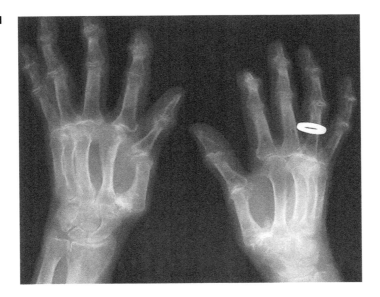

Osteochondritis dissecans (Fig. 3.17)

Caused by local bone necrosis (death of tissue) resulting in loose fragments of bone (loose bodies) in the joint space. The most common site is the knee.

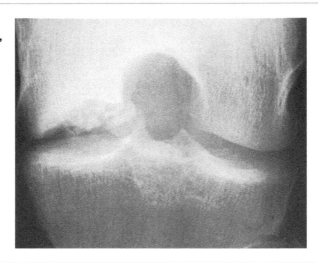

Fig. 3.17 **Osteo-chondritis dissecans, medial condyle of femur.**
(From Sutton 1987.)

Juvenile osteochondritis (Fig. 3.18)

A non-inflammatory condition of epiphyses or centres of ossification. It may be due to poor blood supply causing necrosis.

Radiological signs (late) – increased bone density and fragmentation of the epiphysis. Different names according to site, e.g. Perthes' disease (see Fig. 7.17) – head of femur; Osgood–Schlatter's disease (Fig. 3.18) – tibial tubercle.

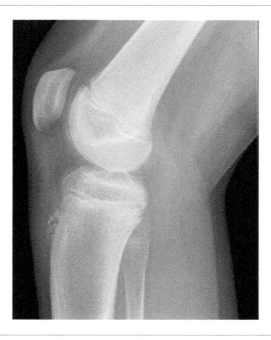

Fig. 3.18 **Osgood–Schlatter's disease, knee.** Note fragmentation of the tibial tubercle with overlying soft tissue thickening.

BONE TUMOURS

Bone cysts (not actual tumours) (Fig. 3.19)

These are cavities in the bone filled with fluid. They may be responsible for pathological fractures.

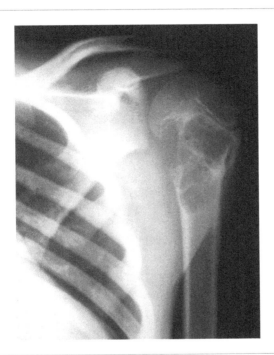

Fig. 3.19 Bone cysts, humerus, with pathological fracture. (Courtesy of Ernest Higginbottom.)

Benign tumours

Radiographically, these have well defined edges and the bone cortex is intact.

Osteoma

A benign tumour of the osteoblasts.

Chondroma
(Fig. 3.20)

A tumour of mature cartilage, the most common sites being the phalanges of the fingers. It may undergo malignant changes.

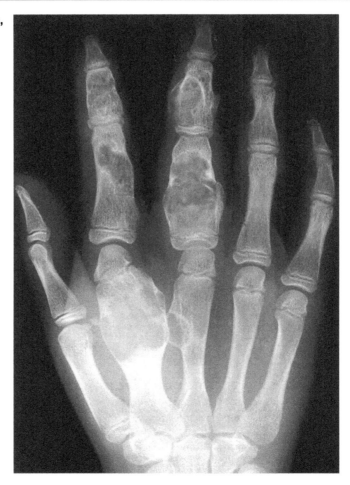

Fig. 3.20 Chondroma, hand. (From Sutton 1987.)

Osteochondroma
(Fig. 3.21)

A tumour of the cartilaginous cells, most common in the 10–25 age group.

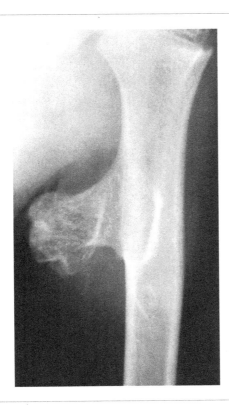

Fig. 3.21
Osteochondroma, humerus.
(From Sutton 1987.)

Osteoclastoma (giant cell tumour)
(Fig. 3.22)

Thought to be a tumour of the osteoclasts, most common in the 20–35 age group. Most common sites are the long bones, particularly round the knee.

Malignant tumours

Radiographically, these have ill-defined edges, destruction of the bone cortex, periosteal reaction and rapid growth. Blood-borne spread is usually to the lungs.

Osteosarcoma (osteogenic sarcoma)
(Fig. 3.23)

A tumour of the osteoblasts, which can occur in any bone but is usually found at the end of a long bone. Most common in male adolescents. Spreads rapidly to patient's lungs.

Radiological signs – area of radio-opacity with periosteal reaction.

**Fig. 3.22 Osteo-
clastoma (giant cell
tumour) of distal
radius.**

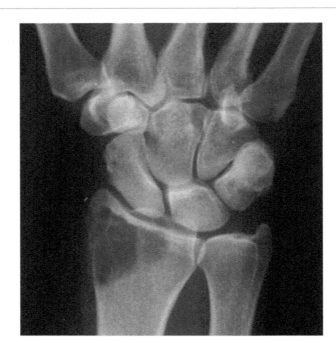

**Fig. 3.23 Osteo-
sarcoma, knee**
(pathology specimen).
(Courtesy of Ernest
Higginbottom.)

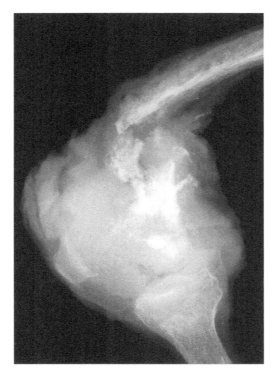

Chondrosarcoma
(Fig. 3.24)

A tumour of cartilage cells, metastasising to the lungs. Most common sites are the pelvis, long bones and round the knee joint.

Fig. 3.24
Chondrosarcoma, femur.
(From Sutton 1987.)

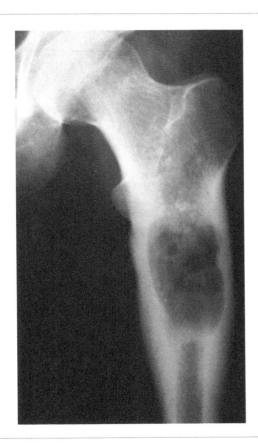

Fibrosarcoma

A rare tumour of fibrous tissue. Most common at the ends of long bones but may occur mid-shaft. Results in bone destruction.

Ewing's tumour

A rare tumour, most common in adolescents. Thought to be a tumour of the reticulo-endothelial cells, metastasising through the bloodstream to the lungs and other bones.

Myelomatosis (multiple myeloma) (Fig. 3.25)

Probably a tumour of the bone marrow, most common in the 60-plus age group. Destroys bone tissue and produces multiple lesions. Pathological fractures are common. Common sites are the spine, skull, ribs, pelvis, upper femur, shoulder girdle and humerus.

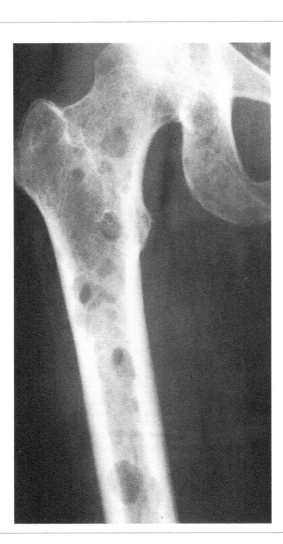

Fig. 3.25 **Myelo-matosis, femur.** (From Sutton 1987.)

Secondary bone tumours (Figs 3.26, Figs 3.27, Plates 2, 3 and 4)

These may occur from a primary tumour of the prostate, breast, bronchus, kidney, stomach or thyroid. They produce simple or multiple, extremely painful, lesions. Common sites are the vertebral bodies, upper ends of long bones, e.g. femur and humerus, pelvis, ribs and the skull. Nuclear medicine techniques will demonstrate metastases that are not demonstrated radiographically in the early stages.

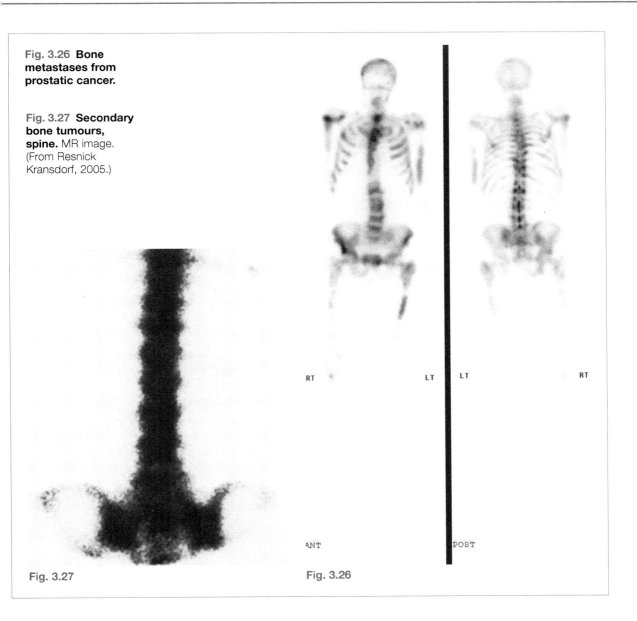

Fig. 3.26 **Bone metastases from prostatic cancer.**

Fig. 3.27 **Secondary bone tumours, spine.** MR image. (From Resnick Kransdorf, 2005.)

RT   LT   LT   RT

ANT   POST

Fig. 3.27   Fig. 3.26

FRACTURES

A fracture is an abnormal break in bone continuity and may be complete or partial.

Causes

Direct trauma
Indirect trauma (usually rotational)
Repetitive strain (stress fracture, e.g. march fracture)
Underlying pathology (tumour, osteogenesis imperfecta, osteoporosis).

Types of fracture

Simple (closed) fracture

This is where the skin surface remains intact and therefore there is no risk of infection.

Compound (open) fracture

This is where the skin surface is broken and there is a direct communication between the body surface and the bone fragments; therefore a risk of infection is present.

Fractures are usually named after the line of the break:

Transverse – horizontally across the bone.

Oblique – obliquely along the bone.

Spiral – spiralling up the bone, usually caused by a twisting movement.

Comminuted – composed of a number of fragments of bone.

Impacted – when one section of bone is pushed into another.

Compression – the bone is crushed; usually occurs in the vertebral bodies or calcaneum.

Greenstick – an incomplete break; occurs in young children.

Depressed – when the bone has been hit by a sharp object; usually occurs in the skull.

Orthopaedic management of fractures

Diagnosis

Signs and symptoms of a fracture may include:

- pain
- swelling
- deformity, e.g. angulation or shortening of a limb
- abnormal movement.

Diagnosis is usually confirmed radiographically

Reduction

The aim of reduction is to realign the bones to as near the normal position as possible and therefore promote faster healing.

Methods available include:

Closed manipulation – usually performed under anaesthetic conditions when the bone ends are moulded together.

Mechanical traction – usually used for fractures of the femur, where the contraction of muscles exerts a strong, displacing force. A weight is attached to the leg and this applies tension, which counteracts the muscular pull, slowly aligning the bones.

Open reduction – a surgical operation where the bones are manipulated directly.

Immobilisation

This ensures that the manipulated fragments of bone maintain their alignment; it therefore encourages faster healing.

Methods available include:

Plaster of Paris bandages – usually used after closed manipulation. Applied wet; when dry, provides a hard, protective cover.

Splints – numerous types available; can be made of aluminium, plastic or polystyrene; tend to be used for fingers.

Screws and plates, pin and nails – inserted during open reduction to internally fix the bone fragments. Used in comminuted fractures and when other methods are difficult to apply, e.g. for the neck of femur.

Rehabilitation

This takes place as soon after immobilisation as possible. The patient is encouraged to move parts of the body to increase the blood supply to the fracture site and therefore quicken healing, for example, in a fractured wrist the fingers are moved and muscle exercises are given.

Stages of healing of fractures

1. A blood clot is formed owing to damaged blood vessels in the medulla, cortex and periosteum.
2. Within 24 hours the haematoma is converted into vascular, fibroblastic granulation tissue.
3. After about 7 days cartilage and osteoid tissue are laid down by the osteoblasts, therefore forming irregular, new bone called provisional callus.
4. Provisional callus is converted into 'normal' bone containing *haversian systems*.
5. After a period of time the bone is moulded by the osteoclasts and osteoblasts to regain its original shape.

Factors influencing the rate of healing

The rate of healing varies from individual to individual and delayed union may result from one or more of the following factors:

Malunion – due to poor reduction.

Infection – common with compound fractures.

Foreign bodies – being present.

Bone fragments – being present.

Poor immobilisation.

Age – generally the older the person the longer the healing owing to the decreased blood supply and slower metabolic rates.

Vitamin and dietary deficiency.

Nonunion occurs if certain tissues (periosteum, muscle, cartilage) are interposed between the ends of the bone.

Common fractures and fracture sites will be discussed after the appropriate bone or joint along with an example of treatment methods used.

Healing of fractures

Radiological evidence of fracture healing
Appearance of callus.

Radiographic signs of bony union (Fig. 3.28)
Visible callus bridging the gap between the bone fragments.
Bone trabeculae continuing across the fracture site.

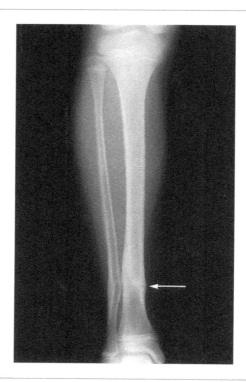

Fig. 3.28 Radiographic signs of bony union, tibia and fibula.
(Courtesy of Ernest Higginbottom.)

Upper limb

4

CHAPTER CONTENTS

HUMERUS (Figs 4.1 and 4.2)

Type	Long bone.
Position	Largest bone in the upper limb.
Articulations	*Head of humerus* with the glenoid cavity of the scapula to form the shoulder joint. *Trochlea* of the humerus with the trochlear notch of the ulna and the *capitulum* of the humerus with the head of the radius to form the elbow joint.
Main parts	**Features of the upper end of the humerus** *Head of humerus* – rounded. *Lesser tuberosity (lesser tubercle)* – anteriorly, the tendon of the subscapularis muscle is attached. *Greater tuberosity (greater tubercle)* – postero-laterally the supraspinatus tendon is attached to the upper aspect, infraspinatus tendon to the middle and the teres minor tendon to the lower, posterior aspect. *Intertubercular sulcus (bicipital groove)* – between the tuberosities. Contains the tendon of the long head of biceps. *Anatomical neck* – adjoining the head. *Surgical neck* – between the upper end and the shaft. **Features of the shaft of the humerus** *Deltoid tuberosity* – for the attachment of the deltoid muscle, located on the antero-lateral surface.

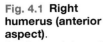

Fig. 4.1 Right humerus (anterior aspect).

A – Lesser tuberosity (tubercle)
B – Greater tuberosity (tubercle)
C – Intertubercular sulcus (bicipital groove)
D – Deltoid tuberosity
E – Lateral border
F – Lateral supra-condylar ridge
G – Lateral epicondyle
H – Radial fossa
I – Capitulum
J – Trochlea
K – Medial epicondyle
L – Coronoid fossa
M – Medial supra-condylar ridge
N – Surgical neck
O – Anatomical neck
P – Head of humerus.

Fig. 4.2 Right humerus (posterior aspect).

1 – Head of humerus
2 – Anatomical neck
3 – Surgical neck
4 – Medial border
5 – Medial supra-condylar ridge
6 – Olecranon fossa
7 – Medial epicondyle
8 – Groove for the ulnar nerve
9 – Trochlea
10 – Lateral epicondyle
11 – Lateral supra-condylar ridge
12 – Spiral groove
13 – Greater tuberosity (tubercle).

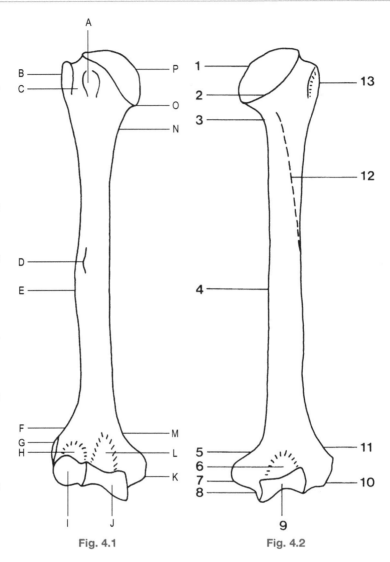

Fig. 4.1

Fig. 4.2

Spiral groove – for the radial nerve.
Medial border.
Lateral border.
Anterior border.
Antero-lateral surface.

Antero-medial surface – in the middle of which is the nutrient foramen.

Posterior surface.

Features of the lower end of the humerus

Lateral epicondyle – above the capitulum.

Medial epicondyle – above the trochlea.

Lateral supracondylar ridge – distal end of the lateral border above the lateral epicondyle.

Medial supracondylar ridge – distal end of the medial border above the medial epicondyle.

Capitulum – rounded; articulates with the head of radius.

Trochlea – pulley-shaped; articulates with the trochlear notch of the ulna. Has a large medial lip which forms the 'carrying angle' (see elbow joint).

Groove for the ulnar nerve – posterior aspect, medial to the trochlea.

Olecranon fossa – posteriorly receives the olecranon process of the ulna when the elbow joint is extended.

Coronoid fossa – anteriorly receives the coronoid process of the ulna when the elbow joint is fully flexed.

Radial fossa – anteriorly receives the head of the radius when the elbow joint is flexed.

Ossification

Primary centre

Shaft – 8th week of intrauterine life.

Secondary centres

Upper end – 3 centres:
    head appears age 6 months;
    greater tuberosity age 1–2;
    lesser tuberosity age 4–5.
    Fuse together age 6.
    Fuse with shaft age 18–20.

Lower end – 4 centres:
    capitulum appears age 1;
    medial epicondyle age 4–6;
    trochlea age 9–10;
    lateral epicondyle age 12.
    Lateral epicondyle, trochlea and capitulum fuse together at puberty.
    Fuse with shaft age 14–16.
    Medial epicondyle fuses with the shaft age 20.

Radiographic appearances of the humerus (Figs 4.3 and 4.4)

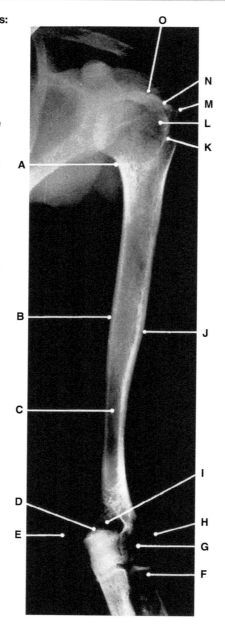

Fig. 4.3 Left humerus: anteroposterior projection. (From Bryan 1996.)
A – Surgical neck
B – Shaft of humerus
C – Medullary cavity
D – Olecranon
E – Medial epicondyle
F – Head of radius
G – Capitulum
H – Lateral epicondyle
I – Olecranon and coronoid fossae
J – Deltoid tuberosity
K – Intertubercular sulcus (Bicipital groove)
L – Lesser tuberosity
M – Greater tuberosity
N – Anatomical neck
O – Head of humerus.

Fig. 4.4 Left humerus: lateral projection.
(From Bryan 1996.)
 1 – Lesser tuberosity
 2 – Intertubercular sulcus (Bicipital groove)
 3 – Radius
 4 – Ulna
 5 – Olecranon
 6 – Trochlea
 7 – Epicondyles
 8 – Supracondylar ridge
 9 – Shaft of humerus
10 – Greater tuberosity
11 – Head of humerus.

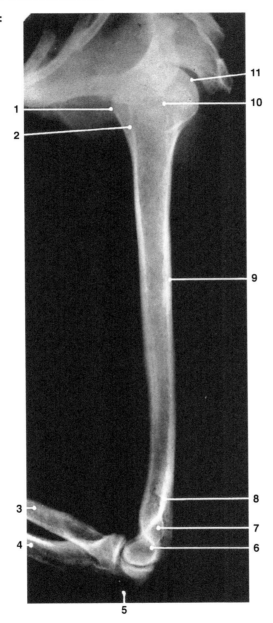

Fractures

Surgical neck
Cause – fall on an outstretched hand. Common in elderly people.
Example of treatment – sling.

Shaft
Usually the middle third.

Spiral
Cause – fall on the hand with a twisting force.
Example of treatment – sling.

Transverse
Cause – fall on the elbow with the arm abducted.
Example of treatment – manipulation under anaesthesia.

Comminuted – transverse or short oblique.
Cause – direct blow on the arm.
Example of treatment – plaster of Paris either to elbow or axilla to mid-forearm, with the elbow flexed.

Pathological – proximal half of the shaft.
Cause – underlying pathology.
Example of treatment – sling; conservative treatment to alleviate pain.

Supracondylar
Cause – fall on the hand with elbow flexed. Distal bone fragment is displaced backwards with the risk of damage to the brachial artery. Common injury in children.
Example of treatment – reduction of the displaced fracture under anaesthesia. Limb immobilised in plaster of Paris with elbow flexed.

Condyles
Cause – relatively uncommon and occurs mainly in children.
Example of treatment – plaster of Paris.

RADIUS (Figs 4.5 and 4.6)

Type
Long bone.

Position
Lateral bone of the forearm.

Articulations
Head of radius with the radial notch of the ulna to form the superior radio-ulnar joint and with the capitulum of the humerus to form part of the elbow joint.
Lower end of the radius with the head of ulna to form the inferior radio-ulnar joint and with the scaphoid and lunate to form part of the wrist joint.

Fig. 4.5 Right radius (anterior aspect).
A – Head of radius
B – Neck of radius
C – Radial tuberosity
D – Oblique line
E – Lateral border
F – Interosseous border
G – Lower end of radius
H – Radial styloid process.

Right ulna (anterior aspect).
I – Ulnar styloid process
J – Medial border
K – Interosseous border
L – Ulnar tuberosity
M – Coronoid process
N – Trochlear notch
O – Olecranon process
P – Radial notch.

Fig. 4.6 Right radius (posterior aspect).
1 – Head of radius
2 – Neck of radius
3 – Radial tuberosity
4 – Lateral border
5 – Interosseous border
6 – Radial styloid process
7 – Ulnar notch.

Right ulna (posterior aspect).
8 – Ulnar styloid process
9 – Head of ulna
10 – Interosseous border
11 – Medial border
12 – Olecranon process.

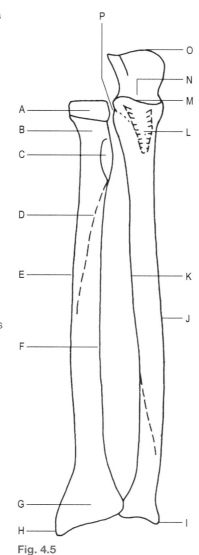

Fig. 4.5

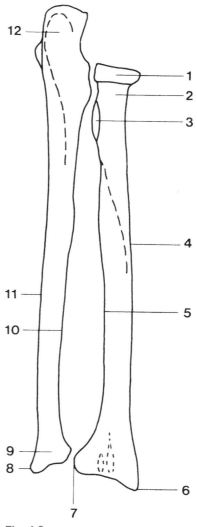

Fig. 4.6

Main parts	**Features of the upper end of the radius**

Features of the upper end of the radius

Head – rounded, with a concave superior surface and an articular circumference.

Neck – narrow portion, inferior to the head.

Radial tuberosity – medial aspect, below the neck, provides attachment for the biceps brachii muscle.

Features of the shaft of the radius

Anterior border.

Posterior border.

Interosseous border – attached to the lateral aspect of the ulna by an interosseous membrane to form the middle radio-ulnar joint.

Anterior surface – the location of the nutrient foramen.

Posterior surface.

Lateral surface.

Features of the lower end of radius

Ulnar notch – located on the medial aspect; articulates with head of ulna to form part of the inferior radio-ulnar joint.

Radial styloid process – prominent process on the lateral aspect which can be palpated.

Distal surface – for articulation with the carpal bones.

Ossification

Primary centre

Shaft – 8th week of intrauterine life.

Secondary centres

2 centres:
> lower end of radius appears age 1;
> head of radius appears age 4–5.
> Head of radius unites with the shaft age 14–17.
> Lower end of the radius unites with the shaft age 17–19.

ULNA (Figs 4.5 and 4.6)

Type

Long bone.

Position

Medial bone of the forearm.

Articulations

Radial notch of the ulna with the head of the radius to form the superior radio-ulnar joint.

Head of ulna with the ulnar notch of the radius to form part of the inferior radio-ulnar joint.

Trochlear notch of the ulna with the trochlea of the humerus to form part of the elbow joint.

(The head of the ulna is covered with an articular disc and therefore does not directly take part in the formation of the wrist joint.)

Main parts

Features of the upper end of the ulna

Olecranon process – postero-superior projection. It can be palpated on the posterior aspect of the elbow joint; it gives attachment to the triceps tendon.

Coronoid process – anterior projection.

Ulnar tuberosity – situated on the anterior surface of the coronoid process; provides attachment to the brachialis muscle.

Trochlear notch – between the coronoid and olecranon processes; articulates with the trochlea of the humerus.

Radial notch – depression on the lateral aspect of the coronoid process; articulates with the head of radius.

Features of the shaft of the ulna

Anterior border.

Posterior border.

Interosseous border – attached to the medial aspect of the radius by an interosseous membrane.

Anterior surface – the location of the nutrient foramen.

Medial surface.

Posterior surface.

Features of the lower end of the ulna

Head – small and rounded.

Ulnar styloid process – prominent process which can be palpated on the medial aspect of the wrist joint.

Ossification

Primary centre

Shaft – 8th week of intrauterine life.

Secondary centres

2 centres:
  lower end of ulna appears age 5–6;
  olecranon appears age 9–11.
  Olecranon unites with the shaft age 14–16.
  Lower end unites with the shaft age 17–18.

Radiographic appearances of the radius and ulna (Figs 4.7 and 4.8)

INSIGHT

Due to the arrangement of the radius and ulna a fracture of the shaft of one of the bones is usually associated with a dislocation or fracture-dislocation of the other bone.

Fig. 4.7 Left forearm: anteroposterior projection.
(From Bryan 1996.)
A – Olecranon
B – Trochlea
C – Coronoid process
D – Ulnar tuberosity
E – Shaft of ulna
F – Head of ulna
G – Ulnar styloid process
H – Triquetral
I – Scaphoid
J – Radial styloid process
K – Lunate
L – Inferior radio-ulnar joint
M – Shaft of radius
N – Radial tuberosity
O – Neck of radius
P – Head of radius
Q – Capitulum
R – Humerus.

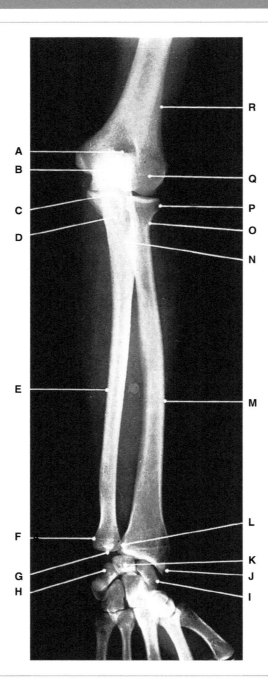

Fig. 4.8 Left forearm: lateral projection.
(From Bryan 1996.)

1 – Epicondyles of humerus
2 – Trochlea and capitulum
3 – Head of radius
4 – Neck of radius
5 – Radial tuberosity
6 – Shaft of radius
7 – Lunate
8 – Scaphoid
9 – Lower end of radius
10 – Head of ulna
11 – Shaft of ulna
12 – Coronoid process
13 – Trochlear notch
14 – Olecranon
15 – Shaft of humerus.

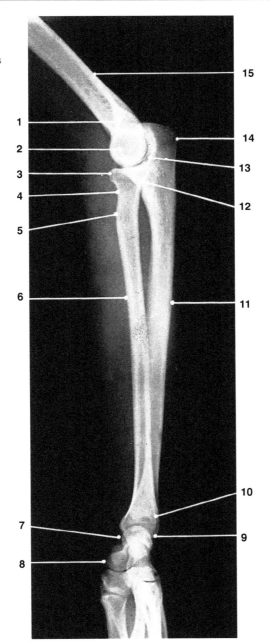

Fractures

Olecranon process   Usually occurs in adults.

Cause – fall on the olecranon process.

Crack without displacement
Example of treatment – plaster of Paris, elbow flexed to 90°.

Transverse with separation
Example of treatment – open reduction and screw fixation, plaster of Paris.

Comminuted
Example of treatment – excision of bone fragments and reattachment of the triceps tendon, plaster of Paris.

Head of radius   Usually occurs in adults.

Cause – fall on the outstretched hand pushes the radial head against the capitulum.

Crack fracture – most common.

Example of treatment – collar and cuff sling.

Comminuted fracture
Example of treatment – excision of radial head.

Mid-shaft radius and ulna   *Cause* – indirect force, e.g. fall on the hand.

Example of treatment – plaster of Paris, elbow to wrist.

Greenstick fracture   Occurs in children.

Cause – direct force, e.g. blow on the forearm.

Example of treatment – plaster of Paris, elbow to wrist.

Monteggia's fracture-dislocation
(Fig. 4.9)

Fracture of the upper third of the ulna with dislocation of the radial head.

Cause – fall on the hand with forced pronation of the forearm.

Example of treatment – plaster of Paris, axilla to head of metacarpals, elbow flexed 90° and forearm supinated; or internal fixation of ulnar fracture by plate and screws or intramedullary nail; plaster of Paris.

Galeazzi's fracture-dislocation
(Fig. 4.10)

Fracture of the lower third of the radius with dislocation of the head of the ulna.

Cause – fall on the hand with a rotational force.

Examples of treatment – plaster of Paris, above elbow to head of metacarpals; or internal fixation of radius by plate and screws.

For fractures of the lower end of the radius and ulna, see wrist joint.

Fig. 4.9 Monteggia's fracture-dislocation.

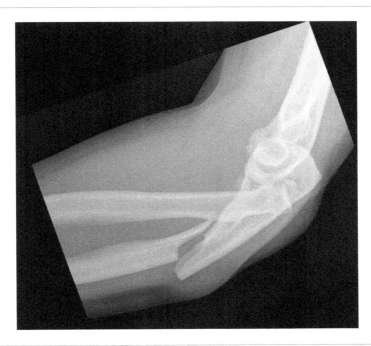

Fig. 4.10 Galeazzi's fracture-dislocation. (From Sutton 1987.)

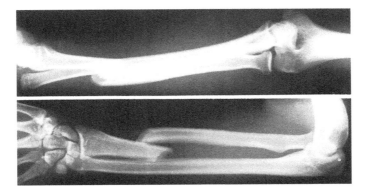

HAND (Fig. 4.11)

Carpal bones

Type	Short bones.
Position	2 rows situated between the radius proximally and the bases of the metacarpals distally.

To remember the position of the scaphoid bones:

Left wrist palmar aspect

Trapezium	Trapezoid	Capitate	Hamate
Under the thumb	Next to the trapezium	Caps the third metacarpal	Has a hook on it
Scaphoid	**Lunate**	**Triquetral**	**Pisiform**
Under the anatomical snuff box	Moon shaped	Under the pisiform	The smallest carpal bone

Articulations	*Scaphoid* with the radius, lunate, trapezoid, trapezium. *Lunate* with the radius, scaphoid, capitate, triquetral. *Triquetral* with the hamate, pisiform, lunate. *Pisiform* with the triquetral. *Hamate* with the 4th and 5th metacarpals, capitate, triquetral. *Capitate* with the 2nd, 3rd and 4th metacarpals, hamate, lunate, scaphoid, trapezoid. *Trapezoid* with the 2nd metacarpal, trapezium, scaphoid, capitate. *Trapezium* with the 1st and 2nd metacarpals, trapezoid, scaphoid.
Ossification	**Primary centres** Appear at the following times of life:

Capitate – 2nd month	Scaphoid – 4th–5th year
Hamate – 3rd month	Trapezium – 4th–5th year
Triquetral – 3rd year	Trapezoid – 4th–5th year
Lunate – 4th year	Pisiform – 9th–12th year.

N.B. The dates at which the carpal bones ossify are subject to considerable variation.

Metacarpal bones (Fig. 4.11)

Type	Miniature long bones.
Position	Distal to the carpal bones.
Articulations	*1st metacarpal* with the proximal phalanx of the thumb, and the trapezium. *2nd metacarpal* with the proximal phalanx of the index finger, the trapezium, trapezoid and capitate. *3rd metacarpal* with the proximal phalanx of the middle finger and the capitate. *4th metacarpal* with the proximal phalanx of the ring finger, the capitate and the hamate. *5th metacarpal* with the proximal phalanx of the little finger and the hamate.

Main parts	*Head* – rounded; articulates with the corresponding proximal phalanx.
	Shaft – anterior border is concave longitudinally.
	Base – expanded; articulates with the appropriate carpal bones. The bases of the 2nd–5th metacarpals articulate with each other.
Ossification	***Primary centre***
	Shaft – 9th week of intrauterine life.
	Secondary centre
	1 centre:
	Base of 1st metacarpal appears age 2–3.
	Head of 2nd–5th metacarpals appear age 2.
	Secondary centre unites with the shaft age 15–19.

Phalanges (Fig. 4.11)

Type	Miniature long bones.
Position	Distal to the metacarpals, forming the fingers.
Articulations	*5 proximal phalanges* with the corresponding metacarpals and the 1st with the distal phalanx of the thumb, the 2nd–5th with the corresponding middle phalanges.
	4 middle phalanges with the corresponding proximal and distal phalanges.
	5 distal phalanges with the corresponding middle phalanges and the proximal phalanx of the thumb.
Main parts	*Head* – expanded; in the distal phalanges supports the tissue of the finger tips.
	Shaft – anterior border is concave.
	Base – expanded; articulates with either the phalanx or the metacarpal proximal to it.
Ossification	***Primary centre***
	Shaft – 8th–12th week of intrauterine life.
	Secondary centre
	1 centre:
	Base of phalanges appears age 2–3.
	Base unites with the shaft age 15–18.

Fig. 4.11 **Right hand (palmar aspect).**

A – Shaft of proximal phalanx of middle finger
B – Shaft of middle phalanx of ring finger
C – Shaft of distal phalanx of little finger
D – Head of 5th metacarpal
E – Shaft of 5th metacarpal
F – Base of 5th metacarpal
G – Hamate
H – Pisiform
I – Triquetral
J – Lunate
K – Capitate
L – Scaphoid
M – Trapezoid
N – Trapezium
O – Shaft of 1st metacarpal
P – Base of proximal phalanx of thumb
Q – Base of distal phalanx of thumb
R – Shaft of 4th metacarpal
S – Shaft of 3rd metacarpal
T – Shaft of 2nd metacarpal
U – Base of proximal phalanx of index finger
V – Shaft of proximal phalanx of index finger
W – Head of proximal phalanx of index finger
1 – Distal interphalangeal joint of index finger (synovial hinge joint)
2 – Proximal interphalangeal joint of index finger (synovial hinge joint)
3 – 2nd metacarpophalangeal joint (synovial ellipsoid joint)
4 – 1st carpometacarpal joint (synovial saddle joint)
5 – 5th carpometacarpal joint (synovial plane joint).

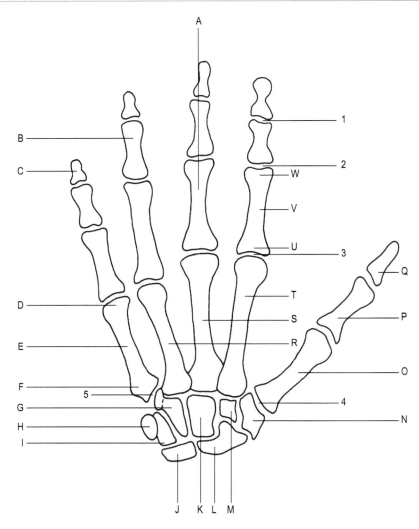

Radiographic appearances of the hand (Figs 4.12, 4.13 and 4.14)

Fig. 4.12 Left hand: dorsipalmar projection.
(From Bryan 1996.)
A – 5th metacarpal
B – Capitate
C – Hamate
D – Triquetrum
E – Pisiform
F – Ulnar styloid process
G – Lunate
H – Scaphoid
I – Trapezium
J – Trapezoid
K – Sesamoid bones
L – Metacarpopha-langeal joint
M – Proximal phalanx
N – Middle phalanx
O – Distal phalanx.

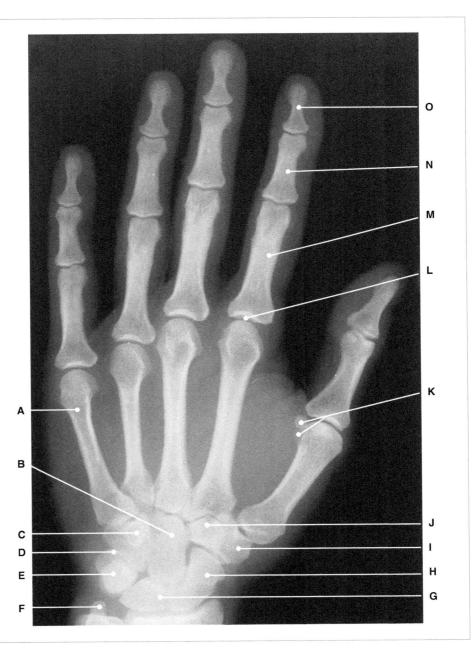

Fig. 4.13 Left hand: dorsipalmar oblique projection. (From Bryan 1996.)
1 – Phalanges
2 – 5th to 2nd metacarpals
3 – Radius
4 – Scaphoid
5 – 1st metacarpal
6 – Phalanges.

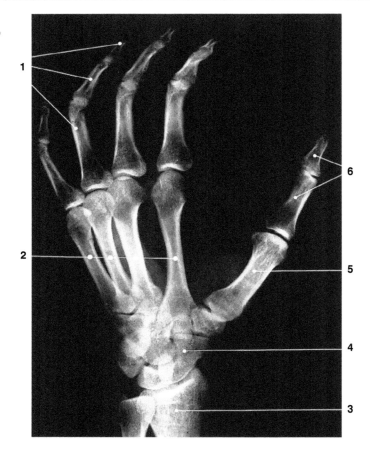

Fig. 4.14 Rheumatoid arthritis: skeletal scintigraphy. Note increased uptake in several proximal and distal interphalangeal joints and the carpi.

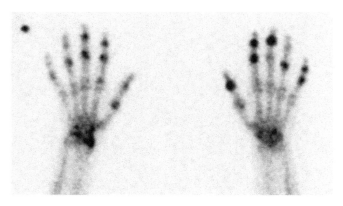

Fractures

Metacarpals	Base, shaft or neck.
	Cause – due to a direct blow.
	Example of treatment – crepe bandage, if no displacement. Plaster of Paris, dorsal slab forearm to fingers if bones displaced.
Phalanges	*Cause* – due to a direct blow.
	Example of treatment – splint for not more than 3 weeks or rehabilitation difficult.

ELBOW JOINT (Figs 4.15, 4.16 and 4.17)

Type	Synovial hinge joint, continuous with the superior radio-ulnar joint.
Bony articular surfaces	Trochlea of the humerus articulates with the trochlear notch of the ulna. Capitulum of the humerus articulates with the head of the radius. The articular surfaces are covered with articular hyaline cartilage.
Fibrous capsule	Attached to the humerus at the level of the epicondyles; extending above the radial and coronoid fossae; incorporating the coronoid and olecranon processes of the ulna and the neck of the radius; blending with the annular ligament of the superior radio-ulnar joint.

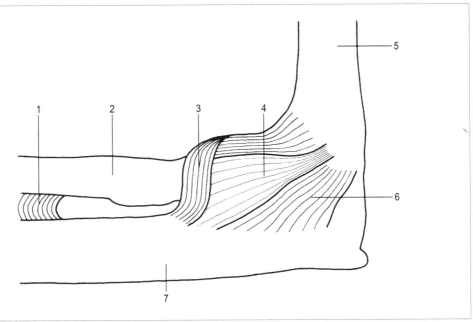

Fig. 4.15 **Left elbow joint (lateral aspect).**
1 – Interosseous membrane
2 – Radius
3 – Annular ligament
4 – Radial collateral ligament
5 – Humerus
6 – Fibrous capsule
7 – Ulna.

Fig. 4.16 Left elbow joint (coronal section).
A – Humerus
B – Trochlea
C – Articular hyaline cartilage
D – Synovial fluid
E – Synovial membrane
F – Ulna
G – Radius
H – Superior radio-ulnar joint
I – Head of radius
J – Annular ligament
K – Fibrous capsule
L – Capitulum.

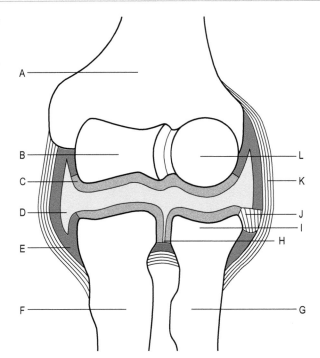

Fig. 4.17 Left elbow joint (sagittal section).
A – Humerus
B – Pad of fat
C – Synovial membrane
D – Articular hyaline cartilage
E – Olecranon process of ulna
F – Radius
G – Annular ligament
H – Synovial fluid
I – Pad of fat
J – Fibrous capsule.

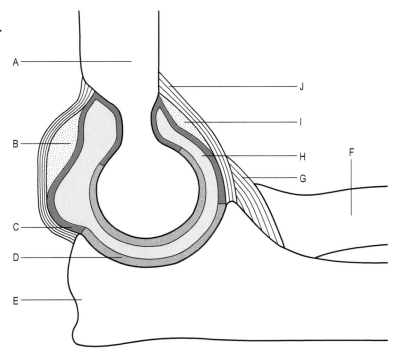

Synovial membrane	Lines the fibrous capsule and the coronoid, radial and olecranon fossae and is continuous with superior radio-ulnar joint. There are pads of fat situated between the synovial membrane and the fibrous capsule above the radial, coronoid and olecranon fossae. The synovial membrane secretes synovial fluid, which lubricates the joint.
Supporting ligaments	*Ulnar collateral ligament* – on the medial aspect of the joint, attached to the medial epicondyle of the humerus and the coronoid and olecranon processes of the ulna.
	Radial collateral ligament – on the lateral aspect of the joint, attached to the lateral epicondyle of the humerus and the annular ligament.
	Annular ligament – surrounds the head of the radius and is attached to the radial notch of the ulna.
Movements	*Flexion* by the biceps, brachialis and brachioradialis muscles.
	Extension by the triceps muscle.
Blood supply	Brachial, ulnar and radial arteries forming an anastomosis.
Nerve supply	Musculo-cutaneous, radial and median nerves.

INSIGHT

The carrying angle is larger in women than men because women have a wider pelvis than men, the angle gets its name from the fact that it allows people to carry items with their arms straight without the forearm catching on the hips.

Carrying angle	Medial angle between the long axes of the humerus and ulna – greater in women than men, the average angle being 163°.

Radiographic appearances of the elbow joint (Figs 4.18 to 4.22)

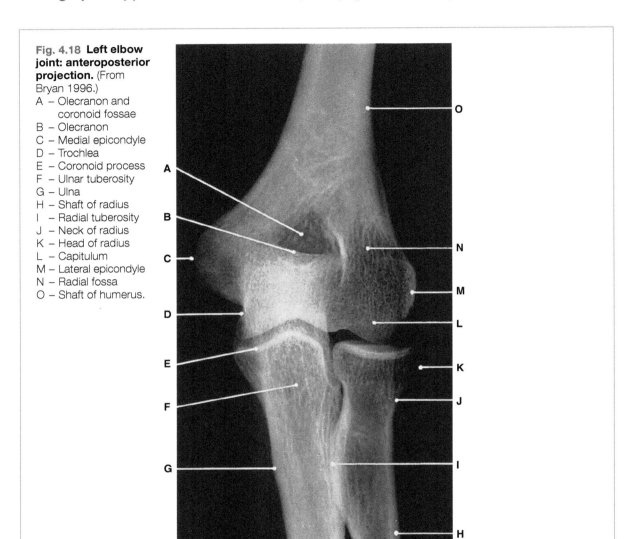

Fig. 4.18 **Left elbow joint: anteroposterior projection.** (From Bryan 1996.)
A – Olecranon and coronoid fossae
B – Olecranon
C – Medial epicondyle
D – Trochlea
E – Coronoid process
F – Ulnar tuberosity
G – Ulna
H – Shaft of radius
I – Radial tuberosity
J – Neck of radius
K – Head of radius
L – Capitulum
M – Lateral epicondyle
N – Radial fossa
O – Shaft of humerus.

Fig.4.19 Left elbow joint: lateral projection. (From Bryan 1996.)
1 – Head of radius
2 – Tuberosity of radius
3 – Shaft of radius
4 – Shaft of ulna
5 – Tuberosity of ulna
6 – Coronoid process
7 – Trochlear notch
8 – Olecranon
9 – Trochlea and capitulum
10 – Epicondyles
11 – Supracondylar ridge
12 – Shaft of humerus.

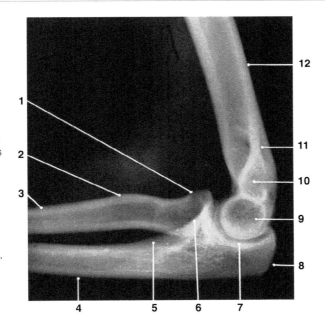

Fig. 4.20 Left elbow joint: oblique projection. (From Bryan 1996.)
A – Olecranon
B – Trochlear notch
C – Radial notch
D – Head of radius
E – Trochlea
F – Capitulum.

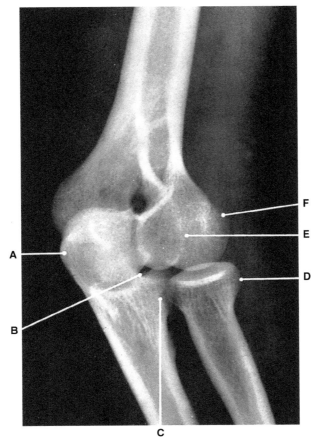

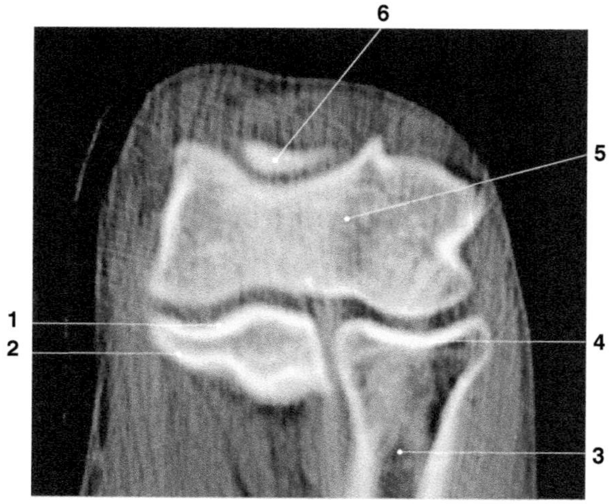

Fig. 4.21 Elbow: CT scan, coronal section. (From Bryan 1996.)
1 – Coronoid process
2 – Ulna
3 – Shaft of radius
4 – Head of radius
5 – Humerus
6 – Tip of olecranon process.

Fig. 4.22 Elbow: CT scan. Note the loose body anterior to the distal humerus (long arrow) and overgrowth of cartilage on the posterior aspect of the radial head (short arrow). (From Resnick Kransdorf, 2005.)

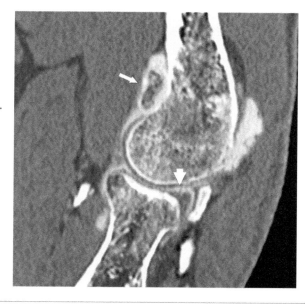

Trauma

Supracondylar fracture

(In children this may be confused with the epiphyses, therefore it is usual to radiograph both elbows for comparison.)

Cause – fall on the hand with the elbow flexed. Distal bone fragment is displaced backwards with the risk of damage to the brachial artery.

Example of treatment – reduction of the displaced fracture under anaesthesia; plaster of Paris with the elbow flexed.

Elbow dislocation

Cause – heavy fall on the outstretched hand. Radius and ulna displaced posteriorly or posteriorly and laterally. Damage to the brachial artery or one of the nerves may occur.

Example of treatment – reduction under anaesthesia. Collar and cuff with the elbow flexed at 90°.

WRIST JOINT (Figs 4.23 and 4.24)

Type

Synovial ellipsoid joint.

Bony articular surfaces

Distal end of the radius with the scaphoid and lunate. Articular disc of the inferior radio-ulnar joint with the lunate and triquetral. The carpal bones are united by interosseous ligaments. The articular surfaces are covered with articular hyaline cartilage.

Fibrous capsule

Attached to the distal end of the radius and ulna, the margins of the joint disc and the proximal aspects of the scaphoid, lunate and triquetral.

Synovial membrane

Lines the fibrous capsule and is separate from the membrane of the inferior radio-ulnar joint. It covers the parts of the bones not covered with articular hyaline cartilage and secretes synovial fluid, which lubricates the joint.

Supporting ligaments

Palmar radiocarpal ligament – from the radius to the scaphoid, lunate and triquetral on the anterior aspect of the joint.

Palmar ulnocarpal ligament – from the ulnar styloid process to the lunate and triquetral on the anterior aspect of the wrist.

Dorsal radiocarpal ligament – from the radius to the scaphoid, lunate and triquetral on the posterior aspect of the wrist.

Ulnar collateral ligament – on the medial aspect of the wrist, attached to the ulnar styloid process and the triquetral and pisiform.

Radial collateral ligament – on the lateral aspect of the wrist, attached to the radial styloid process and the scaphoid.

Intracapsular structures

Articular disc – situated at the distal end of the ulna.

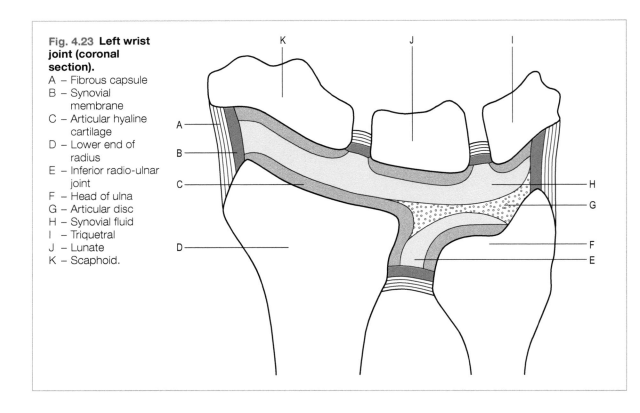

Fig. 4.23 Left wrist joint (coronal section).
A – Fibrous capsule
B – Synovial membrane
C – Articular hyaline cartilage
D – Lower end of radius
E – Inferior radio-ulnar joint
F – Head of ulna
G – Articular disc
H – Synovial fluid
I – Triquetral
J – Lunate
K – Scaphoid.

Movements	*Flexion* by the flexor carpi radialis and flexor carpi ulnaris muscles.
	Extension by the extensor carpi radialis and the extensor carpi ulnaris muscles.
	Abduction by the flexor and extensor carpi radialis muscles.
	Adduction by the flexor and extensor carpi ulnaris.
Blood supply	Radial and ulnar arteries.
Nerve supply	Ulnar, median and radial nerves.

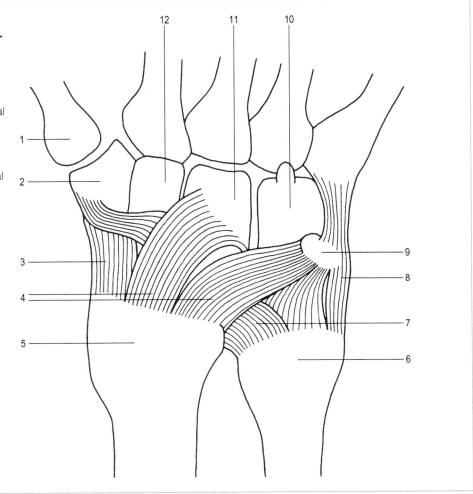

Fig. 4.24 Left wrist joint (palmar aspect).
1 – Base of 1st
  metacarpal
2 – Trapezium
3 – Radial collateral
  ligament
4 – Palmar radiocarpal
  ligament
5 – Lower end of
  radius
6 – Head of ulna
7 – Palmar ulnocarpal
  ligament
8 – Ulnar collateral
  ligament
9 – Pisiform
10 – Hamate
11 – Capitate
12 – Trapezoid.

Radiographic appearances of the wrist joint (Figs 4.25 to 4.30)

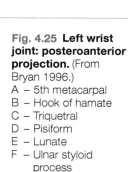

Fig. 4.25 Left wrist joint: posteroanterior projection. (From Bryan 1996.)
A – 5th metacarpal
B – Hook of hamate
C – Triquetral
D – Pisiform
E – Lunate
F – Ulnar styloid process
G – Shaft of ulna
H – Inferior radio-ulnar joint
I – Shaft of radius
J – Radial styloid process
K – Tubercle of scaphoid
L – Trapezium
M – Trapezoid
N – 1st metacarpal
O – Base of 2nd metacarpal
P – Styloid process of 3rd metacarpal
Q – Capitate.

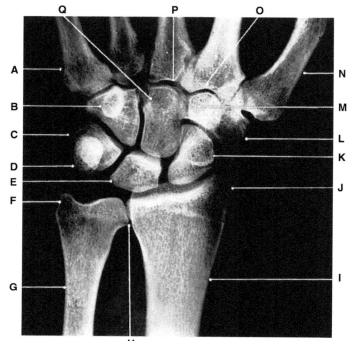

Fig. 4.26 Left wrist joint: lateral projection. (From Bryan 1996.)
1 – 2nd to 5th metacarpal bones
2 – Hamate
3 – Head of capitate
4 – Triquetral
5 – Lunate
6 – Styloid process of ulna
7 – Head of ulna
8 – Ulna
9 – Radius
10 – Styloid process of radius
11 – Scaphoid
12 – Pisiform
13 – Crest of trapezium
14 – Trapezoid
15 – 1st metacarpal
16 – Thenar eminence.

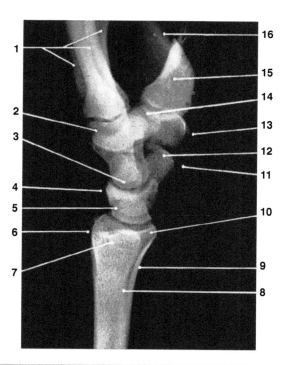

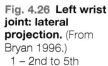

Fig. 4.27 Left wrist joint: posteroanterior oblique projection.
(From Bryan 1996.)
A – Hamate
B – Pisiform
C – Capitate
D – Triquetral
E – Lunate
F – Ulna
G – Radius
H – Scaphoid
I – Trapezoid
J – Trapezium
K – 1st metacarpal.

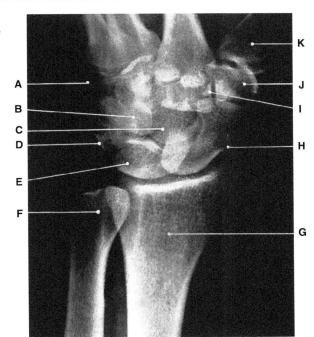

Fig. 4.28 Left wrist joint: anteroposterior oblique projection.
(From Bryan 1996.)
1 – 1st metacarpal
2 – Trapezoid
3 – Trapezium
4 – Scaphoid
5 – Radius
6 – Ulna
7 – Lunate
8 – Pisiform
9 – Triquetral
10 – Capitate
11 – Hook of hamate.

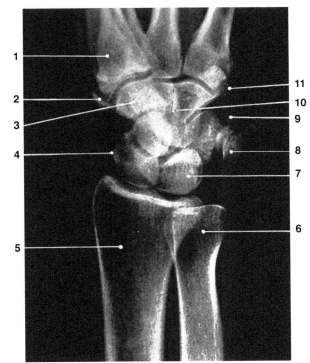

Fig. 4.29 **Wrist: MR scan.** (From Bryan 1996.)
A – Triquetral
B – Pisiform
C – Flexor tendons
D – Scaphoid
E – Lunate.

Dorsal

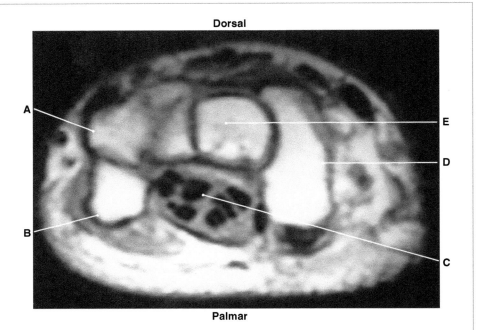

Palmar

Fig. 4.30 **Wrist: MR scan.** Erosion of the radial head (curved arrow) synovitis midcarpal and radiocarpal joints. (From Resnick Kransdorf, 2005.)

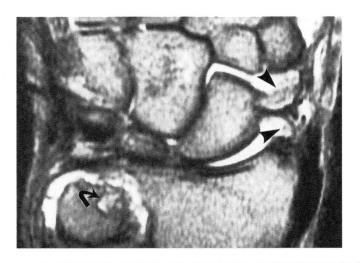

Trauma

Colles' fracture
(Fig. 4.31)

Transverse fracture of the radius with posterior and lateral displacement of the distal fragment. Ulnar styloid process often fractured.

Cause – fall on a dorsi-flexed hand. (Common in elderly women who may have osteoporotic bones.)

Example of treatment – plaster of Paris, below the elbow to the metacarpal necks. Wrist slightly palmar-flexed.

Fig. 4.31 **Colles' fracture.**

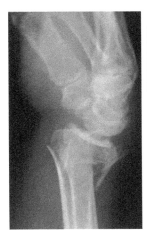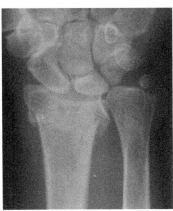

Smith's fracture
(Fig. 4.32)

Transverse fracture of the radius with anterior displacement of the distal fragment.

Cause – flexion injury of the wrist joint (uncommon).

Example of treatment – plaster of Paris, below the elbow to the metacarpal necks. Wrist held in dorsi-flexion.

Fig. 4.32 **Smith's fracture.** (From Sutton 1987.)

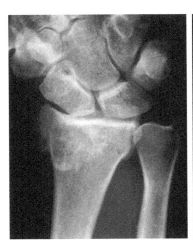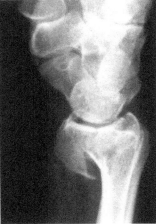

Scaphoid fracture (Figs 4.33 and 4.34)

INSIGHT

If a radiograph of the scaphoid is taken and a fracture is not demonstrated but the pain persists alternative imaging techniques may be required to demonstrate the fracture.

Most common carpal bone to fracture. Often not demonstrated radiographically until 10–14 days following injury. Transverse fracture, middle (waist).

Cause – fall on the dorsi-flexed hand.

Example of treatment – plaster of Paris, upper forearm to head of metacarpals and the proximal phalanx of the thumb.

Fig. 4.33 Scaphoid fractures.

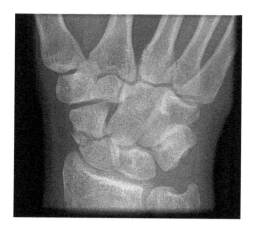

Fig. 4.34 Wrist, scaphoid fracture: radionuclide imaging. Note increased activity in the area of the scaphoid (arrowed). (From Resnick Kransdorf, 2005.)

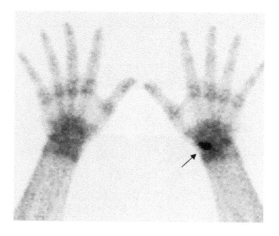

Dislocations

Metacarpophalangeal and interphalangeal joints.

Cause – forced hyperextension of the joint.

Example of treatment – joints strapped in flexion for approximately 1 week.

FIRST CARPOMETACARPAL JOINT

Type	Synovial saddle joint.
Bony articular surfaces	The concave base of the first metacarpal with the convex, superior surface of the trapezium. The articular surfaces are covered with articular hyaline cartilage.
Fibrous capsule	Attached to the perimeter of the base of the first metacarpal and the rough edge round the articular surface of the trapezium. The capsule is thickened dorsally and laterally.
Synovial membrane	Lines the fibrous capsule and is separated from the other carpometacarpal joints. It covers the parts of the bone not covered with articular hyaline cartilage and secretes synovial fluid, which lubricates the joint.
Supporting ligaments	*Lateral ligament* – from the lateral surface of the trapezium to the radial side of the base of the first metacarpal.
	Palmar ligament – an oblique band from the palmar surface of the trapezium to the ulnar aspect of the base of the first metacarpal.
	Dorsal ligament – an oblique band from the dorsal surface of the trapezium to the ulnar aspect of the base of the first metacarpal.
Movements	*Flexion* by the flexor pollicis, opponens pollicis and flexor pollicis longus.
	Extension by the abductor pollicis longus, extensor pollicis brevis and extensor pollicis longus.
	Abduction by the abductor pollicis brevis and the abductor pollicis longus.
	Adduction by the adductor pollicis.
	Axial rotation, a combination of the above movements.
	N.B. Flexion is associated with medial rotation and in full extension the joint is slightly adducted.
Blood supply	Radial arteries.
Nerve supply	Median and radial nerves.

Fractures

**Base of first
metacarpal**

Cause – usually due to a force directed along the long axis of the bone,
e.g. a metacarpal blow as in punching.

Transverse fracture

Example of treatment – firm crepe bandage or plaster of Paris, forearm to
proximal aspect of the first interphalangeal joint.

Bennett's fracture-dislocation (Fig. 4.35)

Oblique fracture extending to the 1st carpometacarpal joint with dislocation
of the thumb.

Example of treatment – plaster of Paris or internal fixation by Kirschner
wires.

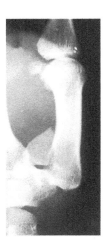

**Fig. 4.35 Bennett's
fracture-dislocation.**
(From Sutton 1987.)

Shoulder girdle | 5

CHAPTER CONTENTS

CLAVICLE (Figs 5.1 and 5.2)

Type Long bone, but it has no medullary cavity and is ossified from a membrane.

Position Runs horizontally from the base of the neck to the shoulder and is subcutaneous throughout.

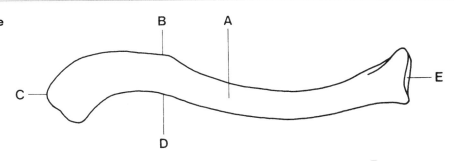

Fig. 5.1 Right clavicle (superior aspect).
A – Shaft
B – Posterior border
C – Acromial end
D – Anterior border
E – Sternal end.

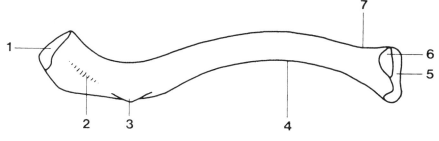

Fig. 5.2 Right clavicle (inferior aspect).
1 – Facet for the acromion
2 – Trapezoid line
3 – Conoid tubercle
4 – Posterior border
5 – Facet for the sternum
6 – Facet for the 1st costal cartilage
7 – Anterior border.

Articulations
The *sternal end* of the clavicle with the clavicular notch of the manubrium sterni to form the sternoclavicular joint.
The *acromial end* of the clavicle with the acromion process of the scapula to form the acromioclavicular joint.

Main parts
Shaft – 'S' shaped.
Sternal end – slightly expanded, quadrangular, medial aspect.
Acromial end – slightly expanded, flattened, lateral aspect.
Facet for the 1st costal cartilage – on the inferior aspect of the sternal end.
Conoid tubercle – on the postero-inferior aspect of the acromial end, coracoclavicular ligament attached.
Trapezoid line – ridge extending laterally from the conoid tubercle, coracoclavicular ligament attached.

Ossification
Primary centres
2 centres in the shaft – 5th week intrauterine life.
Then fuse to form 1 centre at age 45 days.

Secondary centres
1 centre:
Sternal end appears age 18–20.
Sternal end fuses with the shaft age 18–25.

N.B. The clavicle is the first bone to ossify.

Radiographic appearances of the clavicle (Figs 5.3 and 5.4)

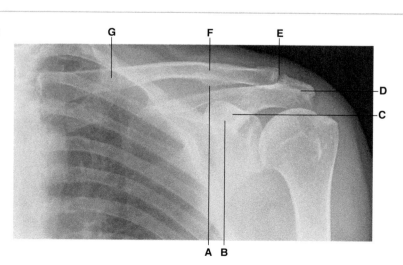

Fig. 5.3 Left clavicle: anteroposterior projection.
A – Conoid tubercle
B – Suprascapular notch
C – Coracoid process
D – Acromion
E – Acromioclavicular joint
F – Lateral one-third
G – Medial two-thirds.

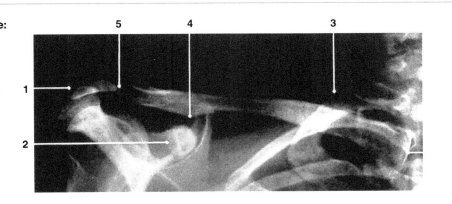

Fig. 5.4 Left clavicle: posteroanterior projection. (From Bryan 1996.)
1 – Acromion
2 – Coracoid process
3 – 1st rib
4 – Conoid tubercle
5 – Acromioclavicular joint.

Fractures

Junction of the middle and outer third

Cause – fall on the outstretched hand.

Example of treatment – reduced by holding the shoulder back by a figure-of-eight bandage.

SCAPULA (Figs 5.5 and 5.6)

Type

Flat, triangular-shaped bone.

Position

Posterior bone of the shoulder girdle, lying on the postero-lateral aspect of the bony thorax extending from the 2nd–7th ribs.

Articulations

Acromion process of the scapula with the acromial end of the clavicle to form the acromioclavicular joint.
Glenoid cavity of the scapula with the head of the humerus to form the shoulder joint.

Main parts

Posterior aspect

Body – triangular in shape.

Spine – narrow ridge dividing the upper third from the lower two-thirds; forms attachment for the trapezius and deltoid muscles.

Supraspinous fossa – depression above the spine for the supraspinatus muscle.

Infraspinous fossa – depression below the spine for the infraspinatus muscle.

Acromion process – broadened, lateral aspect of the spine; on the medial border there is an articular facet for the clavicle.

Superior angle – at the junction between the superior and medial borders.

Fig. 5.5 Left scapula (costal aspect).
A – Scapular notch
B – Superior angle
C – Subscapular fossa
D – Medial border
E – Inferior angle
F – Lateral border
G – Neck
H – Glenoid cavity
I – Coracoid process
J – Acromion process.

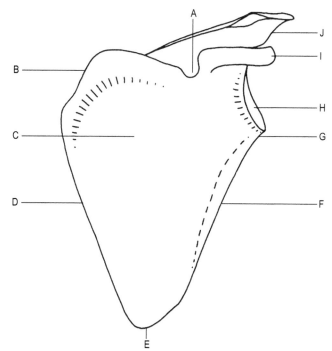

Fig. 5.6 Left scapula (dorsal aspect).
1 – Acromion process
2 – Spine
3 – Lateral border
4 – Inferior angle
5 – Medial border
6 – Infraspinous fossa
7 – Supraspinous fossa
8 – Superior angle
9 – Coracoid process.

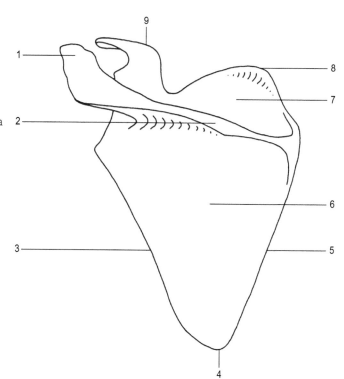

Inferior angle – at the junction between the medial and lateral borders.

Medial (vertebral) border – palpable for most of its length.

Lateral (axillary) border – teres minor is attached below the infraglenoid tubercle.

Spinoglenoid notch – at the junction of the spine and the neck.

Acromial angle – junction of the acromion and spine, posteriorly.

Lateral aspect

Head of scapula – at the lateral angle, formed at the junction of the superior and lateral borders.

Glenoid cavity – 'pear shaped' depression for the head of the humerus on the lateral aspect of the head of the scapula.

Supraglenoid tubercle – superior aspect of the glenoid cavity, tendon of long head of biceps attached.

Infraglenoid tubercle – inferior aspect of the glenoid cavity; provides attachment for the tendon of long head of triceps muscle.

Anterior aspect

Subscapular fossa – large depression for the subscapularis muscle.

Superior border.

Scapular notch – lateral end of the superior border.

Coracoid process – expanded portion, lateral to the scapular notch; provides attachment for the coracoclavicular ligament, short head of biceps and the coracobrachialis muscles.

Ossification

Primary centre

For the body appears near the glenoid cavity – 8th week intrauterine life.

Secondary centres

7 centres:
    coracoid process appears age 1, fuses with body age 15;
    acromion process, 2 centres appear at puberty;
    subarachnoid region appears at puberty;
    lower part of glenoid cavity appears age 14–17;
    medial border appears at puberty;
    inferior angle appears at puberty.
Fuse with body age 20.

Radiographic appearances of the scapula (Figs 5.7 and 5.8)

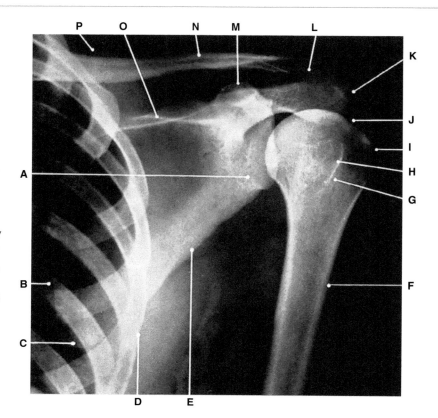

Fig. 5.7 Left shoulder joint and scapula: anteroposterior projection.
(From Bryan 1996.)
A – Glenoid cavity
B – Medial border
C – Inferior angle
D – Chest wall
E – Lateral border
F – Shaft of humerus
G – Intertubercular sulcus (Bicipital groove)
H – Lesser tuberosity
I – Greater tuberosity
J – Head of humerus
K – Acromion
L – Acromioclavicular joint
M – Coracoid process
N – Clavicle
O – Spine of scapula
P – Superior angle.

Fig. 5.8 Left scapula: lateral projection.
(From Bryan 1996.)
1 – Clavicle
2 – Acromion process
3 – Spine of scapula
4 – Head of humerus
5 – Shaft of humerus
6 – Inferior angle
7 – Body of scapula
8 – Ribs
9 – Coracoid process.

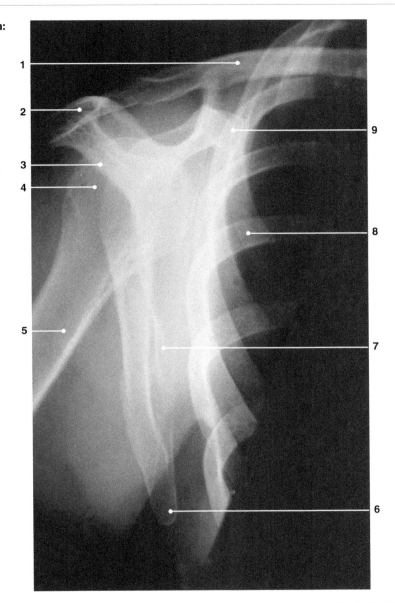

Fractures

Body, neck, acromion and coracoid process

Cause – direct blow.
Example of treatment – sling, for comfort.

SHOULDER JOINT (Figs 5.9 and 5.10)

Type	Synovial ball and socket joint.
Bony articular surfaces	Head of the humerus with the glenoid cavity of the scapula. The articular surfaces are covered with articular hyaline cartilage.
Fibrous capsule	Forms a cylindrical sleeve which is attached medially to the rim of the glenoid cavity and laterally to the anatomical neck of the humerus. The capsule is loose inferiorly to allow movement.
Synovial membrane	Lines the fibrous capsule, encloses the tendon of the long head of biceps and medially is reflected over the glenoid labrum. The membrane secretes synovial fluid, which lubricates the joint.
	Subscapular bursa – lies between the joint and the subscapularis muscle.
	Subacromial bursa – lies between the shoulder joint and the acromion process.
Strengthening ligaments	*Glenohumeral ligaments (superior, middle and inferior)* – from the glenoid cavity of the scapula to the lesser tuberosity and the anatomical neck of the humerus.
	Coracohumeral ligament – from the coracoid process of the scapula to the greater tuberosity of the humerus.

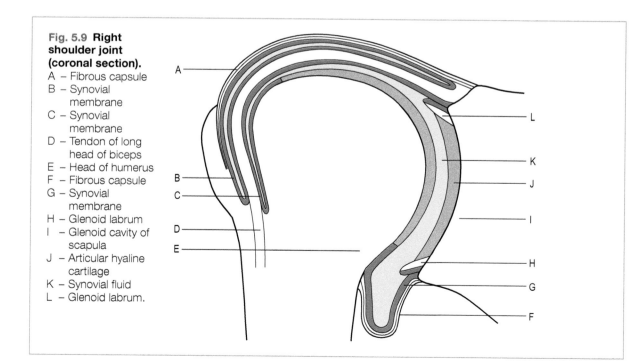

Fig. 5.9 Right shoulder joint (coronal section).
A – Fibrous capsule
B – Synovial membrane
C – Synovial membrane
D – Tendon of long head of biceps
E – Head of humerus
F – Fibrous capsule
G – Synovial membrane
H – Glenoid labrum
I – Glenoid cavity of scapula
J – Articular hyaline cartilage
K – Synovial fluid
L – Glenoid labrum.

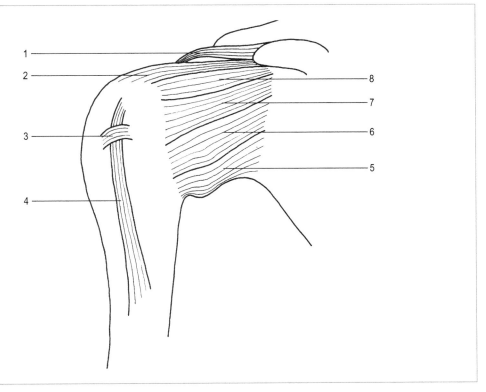

Fig. 5.10 Right shoulder joint (anterior aspect).
1 – Coracoacromial ligament
2 – Coracohumeral ligament
3 – Transverse humeral ligament
4 – Tendon of long head of biceps
5 – Fibrous capsule
6 – Inferior glenohumeral ligament
7 – Middle glenohumeral ligament
8 – Superior glenohumeral ligament.

Transverse humeral ligament – lies between the lesser and greater tuberosities of the humerus and maintains the tendon of the long head of biceps in the intertubercular sulcus (bicipital groove).

Tendons

These reinforce the fibrous capsule, forming the 'rotator cuff':

Supraspinatus tendon attached to the superior aspect of the greater tuberosity of the humerus.

Infraspinatus tendon attached to the middle of the greater tuberosity of the humerus.

Teres minor attached to the lower, posterior aspect of the greater tuberosity of the humerus.

Subscapularis tendon attached to the anterior aspect of the lesser tuberosity of the humerus.

Intracapsular structures

Glenoid labrum – fibrocartilaginous rim round the glenoid cavity to deepen the socket.

Tendon of biceps, long head.

Movements	*Flexion* by the pectoralis major and the anterior fibres of the deltoid.
	Extension by the posterior fibres of the deltoid and teres major, assisted by the latissimus dorsi.
	Abduction by the deltoid.
	Adduction by the pectoralis major and latissimus dorsi, assisted by the teres major.
	Medial rotation by the pectoralis major, anterior fibres of the deltoid, teres major and subscapularis.
	Lateral rotation by the posterior fibres of the deltoid, infraspinatus and teres minor.
	Circumduction – a combination of the above movements.

Blood supply	Branches of the axillary and subclavian arteries.
Nerve supply	Suprascapular, axillary and lateral pectoral nerves.

Radiographic appearances of the shoulder joint (Figs 5.11 to 5.15)

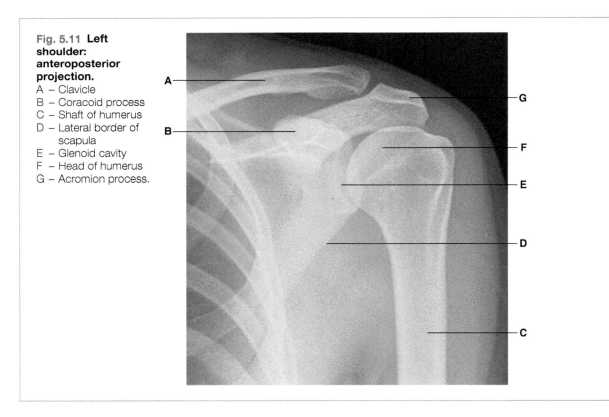

Fig. 5.11 Left shoulder: anteroposterior projection.
A – Clavicle
B – Coracoid process
C – Shaft of humerus
D – Lateral border of scapula
E – Glenoid cavity
F – Head of humerus
G – Acromion process.

Fig. 5.12 **Left shoulder joint: lateral projection.** (From Bryan 1996.)
1 – Coracoid process
2 – Glenoid cavity
3 – Head of humerus
4 – Shaft of humerus
5 – Clavicle.

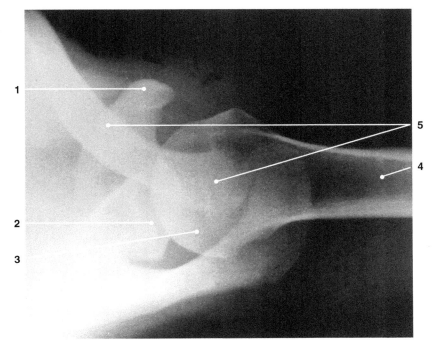

Fig. 5.13 **Shoulder: double contrast CT arthrogram.** (From Bryan 1996.)
A – Head of humerus
B – Air
C – Shoulder joint
D – Contrast medium
E – Scapula
F – Lung
G – Rib.

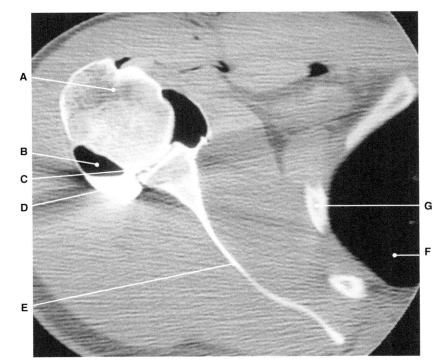

Fig. 5.14 **Shoulder, rotator cuff tear (arrowed). MR scan.** (From Resnick Kransdorf, 2005.)

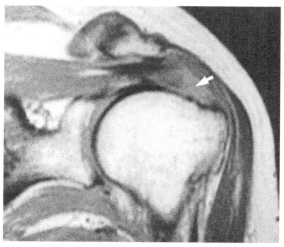

Fig. 5.15 **Shoulder, abnormal glenoid labrum (arrowed). CT arthrotomogram.** (From Resnick Kransdorf, 2005.)

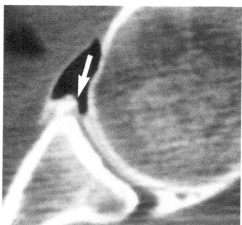

Fig. 5.16 **Shoulder joint, posterior dislocation. CT scan.** (From Resnick Kransdorf, 2005.)

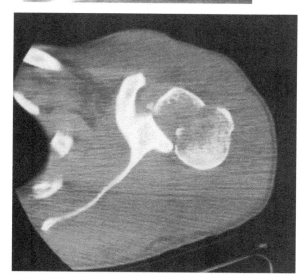

Trauma

Anterior dislocation	*Cause* – fall on the outstretched hand *Example of treatment* – reduction under anaesthetic. Sling for support.
Posterior dislocation (Fig. 5.16)	*Cause* – direct below on the anterior aspect of the shoulder. *Example of treatment* – as for anterior dislocation.
Recurrent dislocation	*Cause* – due to detachment of the glenoid labrum. *Example of treatment* – surgery.

Pathology

Calcification of tendons	Most commonly affects the supraspinatus. *Causes* – acute tendinitis, insignificant trauma and chronic tendinitis; degeneration of the tendon near its insertion following injury. May affect the 'rotator cuff' muscles.

ACROMIOCLAVICULAR JOINT (Fig. 5.17)

Type	Synovial plane joint.
Bony articular surfaces	The acromial end of the clavicle with the medial aspect of the acromion process of the scapula. The articular surfaces are covered with fibrocartilage.
Fibrous capsule	Attached to the lateral end of the clavicle and the medial aspect of the acromion process of the scapula.

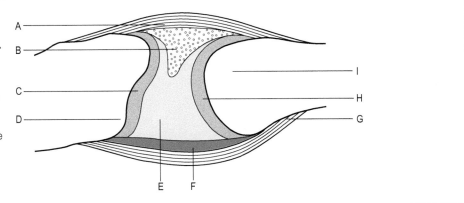

Fig. 5.17 Right acromioclavicular joint (coronal section).
A – Fibrous capsule
B – Articular disc
C – Fibrocartilage
D – Acromion process of scapula
E – Synovial fluid
F – Synovial membrane
G – Fibrous capsule
H – Fibrocartilage
I – Acromial end of clavicle.

Synovial membrane	Lines the fibrous capsule and is reflected over the lateral aspect of the articular disc. The membrane secretes synovial fluid, which lubricates the joint.
Supporting ligaments	*Acromioclavicular ligament* – from the superior aspect of the acromion process to the superior aspect of the clavicle.
	Coracoclavicular ligament – from the coracoid process of the scapula to the conoid tubercle and the trapezoid line of the clavicle.
Intracapsular structure	*Articular disc* – in the upper aspect of the joint, wider superiorly, sometimes absent.
Movements	Gliding.
Blood supply	*Suprascapular artery* – branch of the subclavian artery.
	Thoraco-acromial artery – branch of the axillary artery.
Nerve supply	Suprascapular and lateral pectoral nerves.

Radiographic appearances of the acromioclavicular joint (Fig. 5.18)

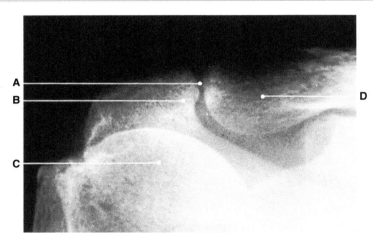

Fig. 5.18 Right acromioclavicular joint: anteroposterior projection. (From Bryan 1996.)
A – Acromioclavicular joint
B – Acromion process
C – Head of humerus
D – Clavicle.

Trauma

Subluxation (partial dislocation)	*Cause* – fall on the shoulder.
	Example of treatment – sling worn for support. Coracoclavicular ligament torn.
Dislocation	*Cause* – fall on the shoulder.
	Example of treatment – internal fixation of the acromion and clavicle with a steel pin, removed after the ligament has healed.

STERNOCLAVICULAR JOINT (Fig. 5.19)

Type	Synovial saddle joint.
Bony articular surfaces	The sternal end of clavicle with the clavicular notch of the manubrium sterni and 1st costal cartilage. The articular surfaces are covered with fibrocartilage.
Fibrous capsule	Attached to the sternal end of the clavicle and the lateral aspect of the manubrium sterni. The capsule thins superiorly and inferiorly.
Synovial membrane	Lines the fibrous capsule and is reflected over the articular disc. The membrane secretes synovial fluid, which lubricates the joint.
Strengthening ligaments	*Anterior and posterior sternoclavicular ligaments.* *Interclavicular ligament* – unites the sternal ends of the clavicles. *Costoclavicular ligament.*
Intracapsular structure	*Articular disc* – divides the joint into 2 distinct parts.
Movements	*Elevation.* *Depression.* *Anterior movement* in a horizontal direction. *Posterior movement* in a horizontal direction. *Circumduction.*

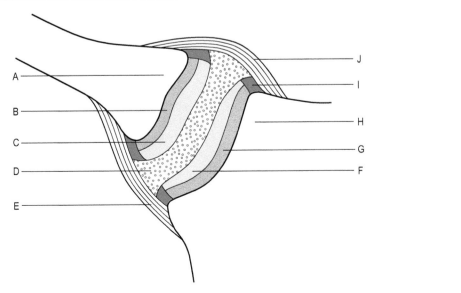

Fig. 5.19 Right sternoclavicular joint (coronal section).
A – Sternal end of clavicle
B – Fibrocartilage
C – Synovial fluid
D – Articular disc
E – Fibrous capsule
F – Synovial fluid
G – Fibrocartilage
H – Clavicular notch of manubrium sterni
I – Synovial membrane
J – Fibrous capsule.

Blood supply   Internal mammary arteries and suprascapular arteries, which are branches of the subclavian artery.

Nerve supply   Anterior supraclavicular nerve.

Radiographic appearances of the sternoclavicular joint (Fig. 5.20)

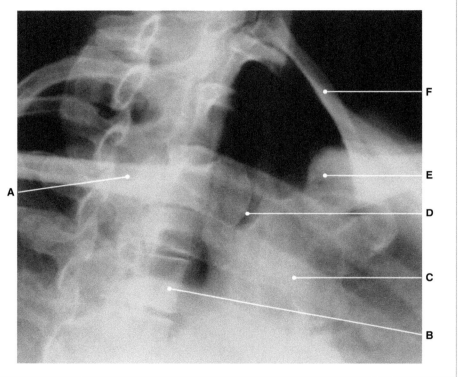

Fig 5.20 Sterno-clavicular joint: anterior oblique projection.
(From Bryan 1996.)
A – Left clavicle
B – Thoracic vertebra
C – Manubrium sterni
D – Left sternoclavicular joint
E – Right clavicle
F – 1st rib.

Trauma

Dislocation
(Fig. 5.21)

Rare.

Cause – fall on the shoulder, forcing the inner end of the clavicle forwards and upwards.

Example of treatment – reduction under anaesthetic; sling.

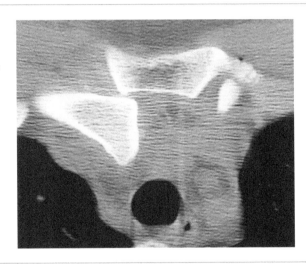

Fig. 5.21 Right sternoclavicular joint, posterior dislocation. CT scan. (From Resnick Kransdorf, 2005.)

Lower limb

CHAPTER CONTENTS

FEMUR (Figs 6.1 and 6.2)

Type

Long bone.

Position

Largest bone of the lower limb forming the thigh.

Articulations

Head of femur with the acetabulum of the hip bone to form the hip joint. *Femoral condyles* with the tibial condyles, and the patellar articular surface of the femur with the posterior aspect of the patella to form the knee joint.

Main parts

Features of the upper end of the femur

Head of femur – rounded, forming two-thirds of a sphere.

Fovea – depression in the head of femur for the ligament of the head of femur.

Neck – narrow portion about 5 cm long joining the head to the shaft; lies at an average angle of approximately 125° (it is more acute in the male than in the female).

Greater trochanter – lies superiorly on the lateral aspect at the junction of the shaft with the neck; provides insertion for the gluteus and piriformis muscles.

Lesser trochanter – inferiorly on the junction between the neck and the shaft, projecting medially; provides insertion of ilio-psoas muscle.

Intertrochanteric line – anterior line, between the trochanters; marks part of the junction between the neck and shaft.

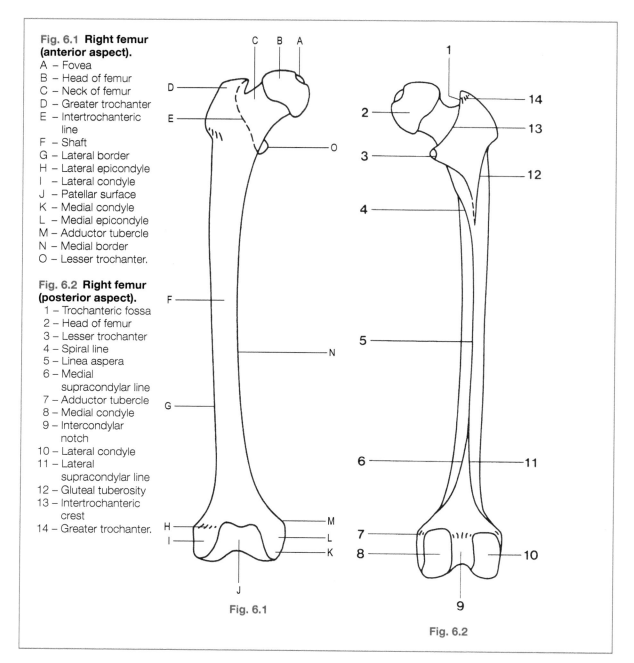

Fig. 6.1 Right femur (anterior aspect).
A – Fovea
B – Head of femur
C – Neck of femur
D – Greater trochanter
E – Intertrochanteric line
F – Shaft
G – Lateral border
H – Lateral epicondyle
I – Lateral condyle
J – Patellar surface
K – Medial condyle
L – Medial epicondyle
M – Adductor tubercle
N – Medial border
O – Lesser trochanter.

Fig. 6.2 Right femur (posterior aspect).
1 – Trochanteric fossa
2 – Head of femur
3 – Lesser trochanter
4 – Spiral line
5 – Linea aspera
6 – Medial supracondylar line
7 – Adductor tubercle
8 – Medial condyle
9 – Intercondylar notch
10 – Lateral condyle
11 – Lateral supracondylar line
12 – Gluteal tuberosity
13 – Intertrochanteric crest
14 – Greater trochanter.

Fig. 6.1

Fig. 6.2

Intertrochanteric crest – posterior crest, between the trochanters; marks part of the junction between the neck and the shaft.

Trochanteric fossa – depression below the medial aspect of the greater trochanter.

Features of the shaft of the femur

Spiral line – posterior aspect, continuous with the intertrochanteric line.

Gluteal tuberosity – lateral surface of the upper end of the shaft, for the gluteus maximus muscle.

Linea aspera – sharp ridge forming the posterior border below the junction of the spiral line and the gluteal tuberosity.

Medial border.

Lateral border.

Anterior surface.

Lateral surface.

Medial surface – the location of the nutrient foramina.

Features of the lower end of the femur

Medial and lateral condyles – fused together anteriorly, separated by the inter-condylar notch posteriorly.

Medial epicondyle – most prominent point of the medial condyle; provides attachment for the tibial collateral ligament.

Lateral epicondyle – most prominent point of the lateral condyle; provides attachment for the fibular collateral ligament.

Intercondylar notch – between the condyles, inferiorly and posteriorly.

Adductor tubercle – above the medial epicondyle; provides attachment for the adductor magnus muscle.

Patellar articular surface – anterior aspect of the lower end of femur, joining the condyles.

Medial supracondylar line – from the adductor tubercle to the linea aspera.

Lateral supracondylar line – from the lateral epicondyle to the linea aspera.

Popliteal surface – flattened triangular area between the supracondylar lines.

Ossification

Primary centre

Shaft – 7th week intrauterine life.

Secondary centres

4 centres:
  lower end appears just before birth;
  head appears age 6 months;
  greater trochanter appears age 4;
  lesser trochanter appears age 13.
  Fuse with shaft age 16–18.

Radiographic appearances of the femur (Figs 6.3, 6.4, 6.5 and 6.6)

Fig. 6.3 Right femur: upper two-thirds; anteroposterior projection. (From Bryan 1996.)
A – Greater trochanter
B – Lesser trochanter
C – Medullary cavity
D – Head of femur
E – Acetabulum.

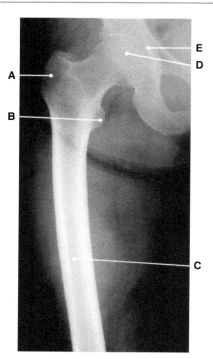

Fig. 6.4 Femur: upper two-thirds; lateral projection. (From Bryan 1996.)
1 – Medullary cavity
2 – Shaft
3 – Lesser trochanter
4 – Femoral neck and greater trochanter superimposed
5 – Head of femur
6 – Acetabulum.

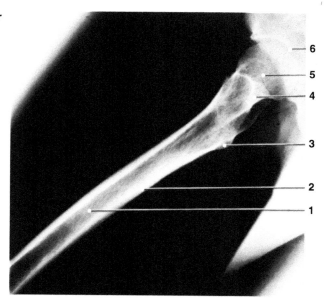

Fig. 6.5 Right femur: lower third; anteroposterior projection. (From Bryan 1996.)

A – Lateral condyle
B – Fibula
C – Tibia
D – Medial condyle
E – Patella
F – Shaft of femur.

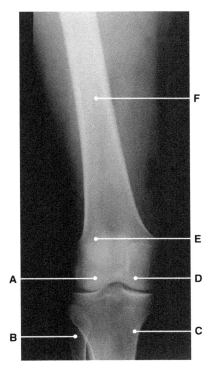

Fig. 6.6 Left knee: lateral projection.
(From Bryan 1996.)

1 – Femur
2 – Intercondylar notch
3 – Condyles of femur
4 – Intercondylar eminence
5 – Superior tibiofibular joint
6 – Fibula
7 – Tibia
8 – Tibial tuberosity
9 – Ligamentum patellae
10 – Apex of patella
11 – Patella
12 – Quadriceps femoris.

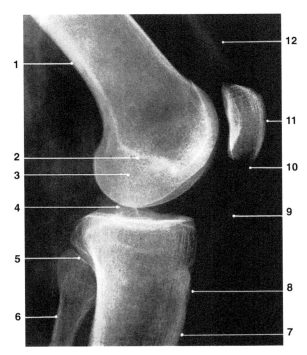

Fractures

Neck of femur

Cause – due to a fall. Common in elderly women.

Example of treatment – reduction under anaesthetic; nail inserted, e.g. Smith–Peterson.

Intertrochanteric fracture

Cause – due to a fall. Common in elderly women.

Example of treatment – reduction under anaesthetic; nails and plate inserted.

Shaft of femur

Fracture pattern variable.

Cause – due to severe violence, e.g. a road traffic accident.

Example of treatment – traction using a Thomas' splint.

Pathological fracture

Shaft of femur.

Cause – bone disease, e.g. metastases.

Example of treatment – internal fixation by an intramedullary nail.

Supracondylar

Cause – due to direct violence. Damage to the popliteal artery or major nerves may occur.

Example of treatment – reduction under anaesthetic; traction using a Thomas' splint.

Stress fracture (Figs 6.7 and 6.8)

Cause – due to prolonged exercise, e.g. athletics, ballet.

Example of treatment – resting the affected area, a plaster cast may be required.

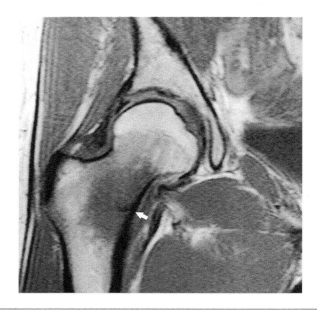

Fig. 6.7 **Right femoral neck, stress fracture (arrowed). MR scan.** (From Resnick Kransdorf, 2005.)

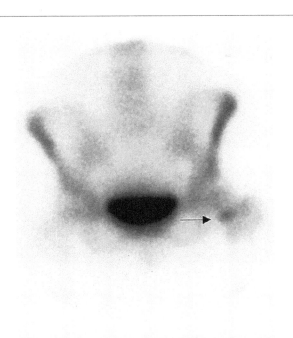

Fig. 6.8 Left femoral neck, stress fracture (arrowed). Radionuclide imaging. (From Resnick Kransdorf, 2005.)

PATELLA (Figs 6.9 and 6.10)

Type	Sesamoid bone.
Position	Anterior to the lower end of the femur.
Articulation	Facets of the patella with the femoral condyles to form part of the knee joint.
Main parts	*Base* – superior aspect, attached to quadriceps femoris by the suprapatellar tendon. *Apex* – inferior aspect, attached by the patellar ligament to the tibial tuberosity. *Facet for the lateral condyle of the femur* – large, on the posterior aspect of the bone. *Facet for the medial condyle of the femur* – small, on the posterior aspect of the bone.

Ossification	**Primary centre**
	Appears age 3–6.
	    Ossification is complete at puberty.
	    N.B. A bipartite or tripartite patella may be seen radiographically in some patients.

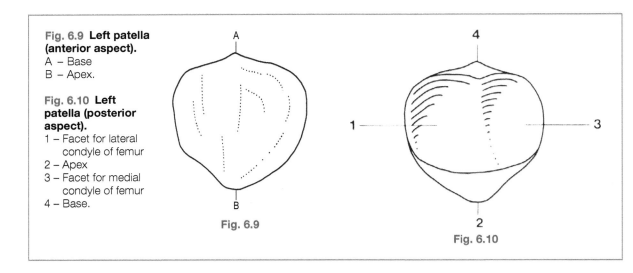

Fig. 6.9 **Left patella (anterior aspect).**
A – Base
B – Apex.

Fig. 6.10 **Left patella (posterior aspect).**
1 – Facet for lateral condyle of femur
2 – Apex
3 – Facet for medial condyle of femur
4 – Base.

Fig. 6.9

Fig. 6.10

Radiographic appearances of the patella (Figs 6.11 and 6.12)

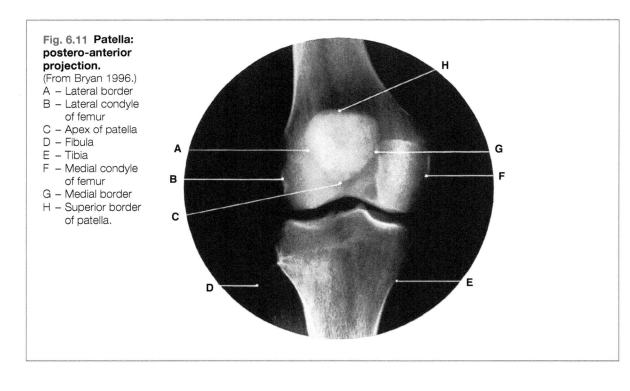

Fig. 6.11 **Patella: postero-anterior projection.**
(From Bryan 1996.)
A – Lateral border
B – Lateral condyle of femur
C – Apex of patella
D – Fibula
E – Tibia
F – Medial condyle of femur
G – Medial border
H – Superior border of patella.

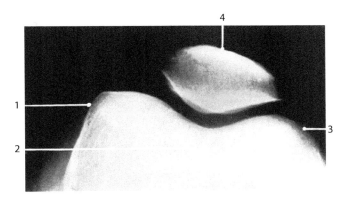

Fig. 6.12 Patella: infero-superior ('skyline') projection. (From Bryan 1996.)
1 – Medial condyle of femur
2 – Femur
3 – Lateral condyle of femur
4 – Patella.

Fractures

Horizontal	*Cause* – sudden, violent contraction of the quadriceps femoris muscle, e.g. due to a stumble. *Examples of treatment* – internal fixation by a screw or excision of the patella.
Crack	*Cause* – direct blow; not to be confused with a bipartite patella, which has 'clean' edges. *Example of treatment* – plaster of Paris (groin to ankle) for 3 weeks.
Comminuted	*Cause* – direct blow. *Example of treatment* – excision of the patella at operation.

TIBIA (Figs 6.13 and 6.14)

Type	Long bone.
Position	Medial bone of the lower limb.
Articulations	*Tibial condyles* with the femoral condyles to form the knee joint. *Articular facet* on the lateral condyle of the tibia with the head of fibula to form the superior tibiofibular joint. *Lower end of tibia* with the talus to form part of the ankle joint. *Fibular notch* of the tibia with the lower end of fibula to form the inferior tibiofibular joint.

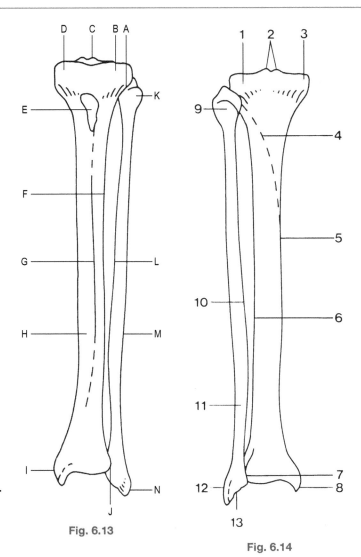

Fig. 6.13 Left tibia (anterior aspect).
A – Fibular facet
B – Lateral condyle
C – Tubercles of the intercondylar eminence
D – Medial condyle
E – Tibial tuberosity
F – Interosseous border
G – Anterior border
H – Medial surface
I – Medial malleolus
J – Fibular notch.
Left fibula (anterior aspect).
K – Head of fibula
L – Interosseous border
M – Lateral surface
N – Lateral malleolus.

Fig. 6.14 Left tibia (posterior aspect).
1 – Lateral condyle
2 – Tubercles of the intercondylar eminence
3 – Medial condyle
4 – Soleal line
5 – Medial border
6 – Interosseous border
7 – Fibular notch
8 – Medial malleolus.
Left fibula (posterior aspect).
9 – Head of fibula
10 – Interosseous border
11 – Posterior border
12 – Lateral malleolus
13 – Malleolar fossa.

Fig. 6.13

Fig. 6.14

Main parts

Features of the upper end of tibia

Tubercles of the intercondylar eminence – on the superior aspect of the tibia between the articular surfaces.

Medial condyle – medial part of the upper end, larger of the 2 condyles.

Lateral condyle – lateral part of the upper end.

Articular facet – on the postero-lateral aspect of the lateral condyle for the head of fibula.

Tibial tuberosity – anterior aspect; can be palpated 2.5 cm below the condyles; forms attachment for the patellar ligament.

Features of the shaft of tibia

Soleal line – 'horseshoe-shaped' oblique line; posterior aspect of the shaft which receives the soleus muscle.

Anterior border – subcutaneous and easily palpated.

Medial border.

Interosseous border – attached to the medial aspect of the fibula by an interosseous membrane to form the middle tibiofibular joint.

Medial surface.

Lateral surface.

Posterior surface – nutrient foramen is situated inferior to the soleal line.

Features of the lower end of the tibia

Medial malleolus – palpable feature at the medial aspect of the lower end.

Fibular notch – lateral aspect of the lower end, for the lower end of the fibula.

Inferior articular surface – concavo-convex for articulation with the superior surface of the talus.

Anterior surface.

Posterior surface.

Ossification

Primary centre

Shaft – 7th week intrauterine life.

Secondary centres

2 centres:
upper end appears just before or after birth;
lower end appears age 1.
Lower end fuses with the shaft age 15–17.
Upper end fuses with the shaft age 16–18.

FIBULA (Figs 6.13 and 6.14)

Type   Long bone.

Position   Lateral bone of the lower leg.

Articulations   *Head of fibula* with the articular facet of the lateral condyle of the tibia to form the superior tibiofibular joint.
Lower end of fibula with the fibular notch of the tibia to form the inferior tibiofibular joint.
Lateral malleolus of the fibula with the talus to form part of the ankle joint.

Main parts   ### Features of the upper end of the fibula

Head – rounded upper aspect; can be palpated 2.5 cm inferior to the lateral aspect of the knee joint.

Styloid process – pointed, upper part of the head.

Neck – narrow area below the head; common fracture site.

Features of the shaft of fibula
Anterior border.

Posterior border.

Interosseous border – connected to the lateral aspect of the tibia by an interosseous membrane to form the middle tibiofibular joint.

Nutrient foramen.

Features of the lower end of fibula
Lateral malleolus – lateral aspect of the lower end; easily palpated.

Articular facet – on medial aspect of the lateral malleolus.

Malleolar fossa – depression on the posterior part of the medial aspect of the lower end; provides attachment for part of the lateral ligament at the ankle joint.

Ossification

Primary centre
Shaft – 8th week intrauterine life.

Secondary centres
2 centres:
  lower end appears age 1;
  upper end appears age 3–4.
  Lower end fuses with shaft age 15–17.
  Upper end fuses with shaft age 17–19.

Radiographic appearances of the tibia and fibula (Figs 6.15 and 6.16)

Fig. 6.15 Left tibia and fibula: anteroposterior projection.
A – Tubercles of intercondylar eminence
B – Medial condyle
C – Tibial tubercle
D – Interosseous borders
E – Tibia
F – Medullary cavity
G – Medial border
H – Medial malleolus
I – Talus
J – Lateral malleolus
K – Inferior tibiofibular joint
L – Shaft of fibula
M – Neck of fibula
N – Head of fibula
O – Superior tibiofibular joint
P – Lateral condyle
Q – Femur.

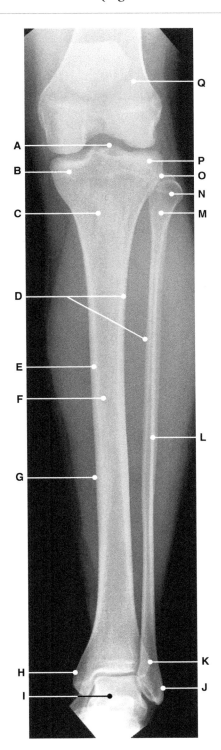

Fig. 6.16 Left tibia and fibula: lateral projection.
1 – Condyles of femur
2 – Head of fibula
3 – Shaft of fibula
4 – Calcaneus
5 – Talus
6 – Ankle joint
7 – Shaft of tibia
8 – Anterior border
9 – Tibial tubercle
10 – Knee joint
11 – Patella.

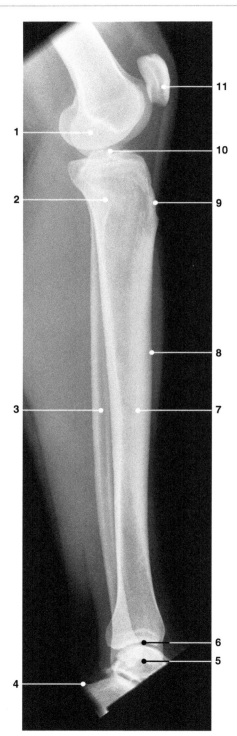

Fractures

Shaft of tibia and/or fibula

Cause – usually motorcycle accidents.

Example of treatment – reduction under anaesthetic; plaster of Paris below hip to foot. Internal fixation may be required.

Tibial condyle (Fig. 6.17)

Cause – abduction of the tibia on the femur, e.g. car bumper striking a pedestrian.

Example of treatment – bed rest for 3–6 weeks, knee in removable plaster; physiotherapy.

Fig. 6.17 Tibial condyle fracture (arrowheads). MR scan. Note the horizontal tear of the lateral meniscus (arrowed). (From Resnick Kransdorf, 2005.)

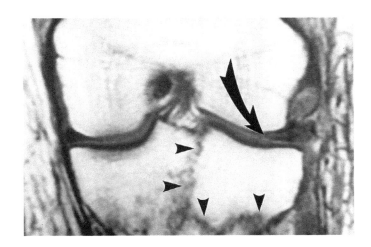

FOOT

Tarsal bones (Fig. 6.18)

Type Short bones.

Position Two rows situated between the tibia proximally and the bases of the metatarsals distally.

INSIGHT

To remember the tarsal bones:
Right foot dorsal aspect

Medial cuneiform	Intermediate cuneiform	Lateral cuneiform	Cuboid
Nearest the midline	The middle cuneiform	The cuneiform nearest the cuboid	Cube shaped
Navicular			
Boat shaped			
Talus			Calcaneus
Forms the ankle joint	(talus means ankle)		Largest tarsal bone

Fig. 6.18 Right foot (dorsal aspect).

A – Shaft of distal phalanx of great toe
B – Shaft of proximal phalanx of great toe
C – Shaft of 1st metatarsal
D – Medial cuneiform
E – Intermediate cuneiform
F – Lateral cuneiform
G – Navicular
H – Talus
I – Calcaneus
J – Cuboid
K – Base of 5th metatarsal
L – Shaft of 5th metatarsal
M – Head of 5th metatarsal
N – Shaft of proximal phalanx of 5th toe
O – Shaft of middle phalanx of 4th toe
P – Head of distal phalanx of 3rd toe
1 – Interphalangeal joint of great toe (synovial hinge joint)
2 – 1st metatarso-phalangeal joint (synovial ellipsoid joint)
3 – 5th distal interpha-langeal joint (synovial hinge joint)
4 – 2nd proximal inter-phalangeal joint (synovial hinge joint).

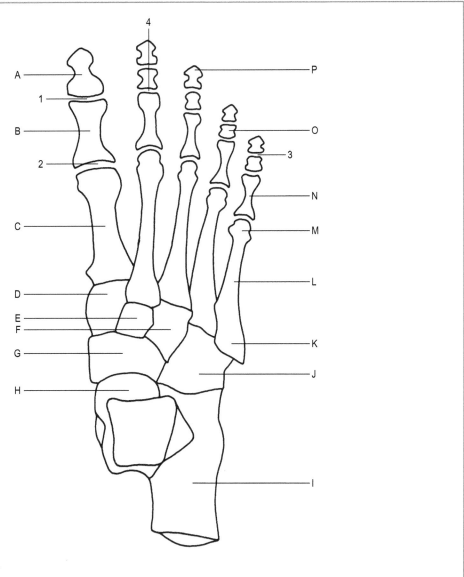

Articulations

Talus with the tibia, fibula, calcaneus, navicular.
Calcaneus with the talus, cuboid.
Navicular with the talus, cuboid, medial cuneiform, intermediate cuneiform, lateral cuneiform.
Cuboid with the calcaneus, navicular, lateral cuneiform, 4th metatarsal, 5th metatarsal.
Lateral cuneiform with the navicular, cuboid, intermediate cuneiform, 2nd, 3rd and 4th metatarsals.

Intermediate cuneiform with the navicular, lateral cuneiform, medial cuneiform, 2nd metatarsal.

Medial cuneiform with the navicular, intermediate cuneiform, 1st and 2nd metatarsals.

Individual bones

Proximal row

Talus

Head – distal end of the bone; articulates with the navicular.

Neck – narrowed section posterior to the head.

Body – cuboidal in shape.

Trochlear articular surface – convex, upper aspect of the body.

Inferior surface – carries the anterior, posterior and middle articular facets for articulation with the calcaneus to form the talocalcanean joint.

Sulcus tali – deep groove between the middle and posterior articular facets.

Calcaneus

Largest of the tarsal bones, situated inferiorly and slightly laterally to the talus.

Superior surface – has three facets (anterior, middle and posterior) for the talus.

Inferior surface – slightly concave.

Posterior surface – large and convex; provides insertion for the Achilles tendon.

Medial surface – concave; the sustentaculum tali projects from the anterosuperior aspect.

Anterior surface – small; articulates with the cuboid.

Sulcus calcanei – lies between the middle and posterior facets.

Lateral surface – flattened except for the peroneal tubercle.

Radiographic appearances of the calcaneus (Fig. 6.19)

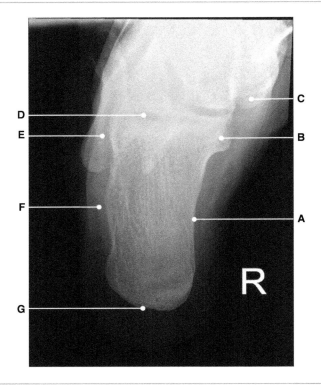

Fig. 6.19 **Right calcaneus: axial projection.**
A – Medial surface
B – Sustentaculum tali
C – Medial malleolus
D – Posterior talocalcanean articulation
E – Lateral malleolus
F – Lateral surface
G – Posterior surface.

Distal row

Navicular
Roughly disc-shaped.

Proximal surface – concave.

Distal surface – convex, and carries 3 facets which articulate with the 3 cuneiform bones.

Cuneiform bones
Wedge-shaped bones.
No parts of significance.

Cuboid
Flattened, six-sided bone.

Lateral and inferior (plantar) surfaces – have a deep groove for the peroneus longus tendon.

Ossification

Primary centres
1 per tarsal bone

Calcaneus – 3rd–4th month intrauterine life.

Talus – 6th month intrauterine life.

Cuboid – 9th month intrauterine life.

Lateral cuneiform – age 1.

Medial cuneiform – age 2.

Intermediate cuneiform – age 3.

Navicular – age 3.

Secondary centres

Calcaneus – Posterior aspect of the calcaneus appears age 6–8. Fuses at puberty.

Talus – May have a secondary centre at the posterior aspect.

N.B. If the centre does not fuse it forms a bone – the os trigonum.

Metatarsal bones (Fig. 6.18)

Type	Miniature long bones.
Position	Distal to the tarsal bones.
Articulations	*The head of the metatarsals* with the phalanges to form the metatarsophalangeal joints.
	The base of the metatarsals with the tarsal bones to form the tarsometatarsal joints.
	1st metatarsal with the proximal phalanx of the hallux and the medial cuneiform.
	2nd metatarsal with the proximal phalanx of the 2nd toe, the medial, intermediate and lateral cuneiform bones.
	3rd metatarsal with the proximal phalanx of the 3rd toe and the lateral cuneiform.
	4th metatarsal with the proximal phalanx of the 4th toe, the lateral cuneiform and the cuboid.
	5th metatarsal with the proximal phalanx of the 5th toe and the cuboid.
	The bases of the 2nd–5th metatarsals with the adjacent metatarsal.
Main parts	*Head* – rounded; articulates with the corresponding proximal phalanx.
	Shaft – plantar aspect concave, dorsal aspect convex.
	Base – expanded; articulates with the appropriate tarsal bone(s).
First metatarsal	Short and thick.
	Articular facets – 2 on the plantar aspect of the head for the sesamoid bones.

Second metatarsal	Longest.
Fifth metatarsal	*Tuberosity* – projects laterally from the base.

Ossification	**Primary centre**
	Shaft – 9th–10th week of intrauterine life.
	
	Secondary centre
	1 centre:
	    base of 1st metatarsal appears age 3.
	    Heads of 2nd–5th metatarsals appear age 3–4.
	    Secondary centre unites with the shaft age 17–20.

Phalanges (Fig. 6.18)

Type	Miniature long bones.
Position	Distal to the metatarsals, forming the toes.
Articulations	*The base of the phalanx* with the metatarsal to form the metatarsophalangeal joints. *With each other* to form the interphalangeal joints. *5 proximal phalanges* with the corresponding metatarsal; the 1st with the distal phalanx of the hallux, and the 2nd–5th with the corresponding middle phalanx. *4 middle phalanges* with the corresponding proximal and distal phalanges. *5 distal phalanges* with the corresponding middle phalanges and the proximal phalanx of the hallux.
Main parts	*Head* – expanded. *Shaft* – plantar aspect is concave. *Base* – expanded; articulates with either the phalanx or the metatarsal proximal to it.

Ossification	**Primary centre**
	Shaft – 9th–15th week of intrauterine life.
	
	Secondary centre
	1 centre:
	    base of phalanges appears age 2–8.
	    Base unites with the shaft age 18.

Arches of the foot	*Medial longitudinal arch* – formed by the calcaneus, talus, navicular, 3 cuneiform bones and 1st, 2nd and 3rd metatarsals; is higher than the lateral longitudinal arch. *Lateral longitudinal arch* – formed by the calcaneus, cuboid and the 4th and 5th metatarsals.

Radiographic appearances of the foot (Figs 6.20, 6.21 and 6.22)

Fig. 6.20 **Right foot: dorsiplantar projection.**
A – Head of distal phalanx
B – Base of proximal phalanx
C – Medial and lateral sesamoid bones
D – 1st tarsometatarsal joint
E – Navicular
F – Talus
G – Cuboid
5th metatarsal bone:
H – Base
I – Shaft
J – Head.

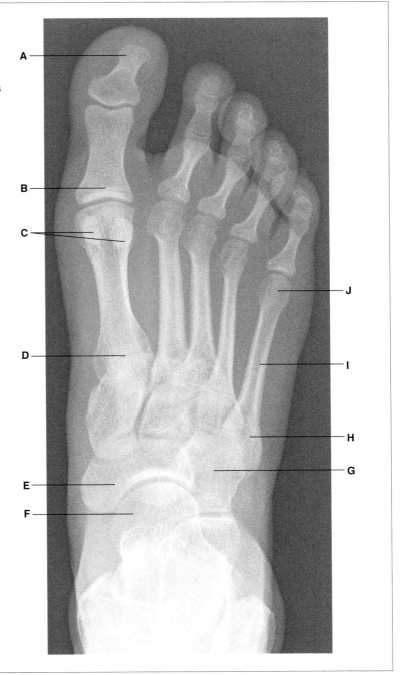

Fig. 6.21 Right foot: dorsiplantar oblique projection.
(From Bryan 1996.)
1 – Distal phalanx
2 – 1st metatarsal bone
3 – Medial cuneiform
4 – Intermediate cuneiform
5 – Navicular
6 – Talus
7 – Ankle joint
8 – Tibia
9 – Fibula
10 – Calcaneus
11 – Cuboid
12 – Base of 5th metatarsal bone
13 – Lateral cuneiform
14 – 5th metatarsal bone.

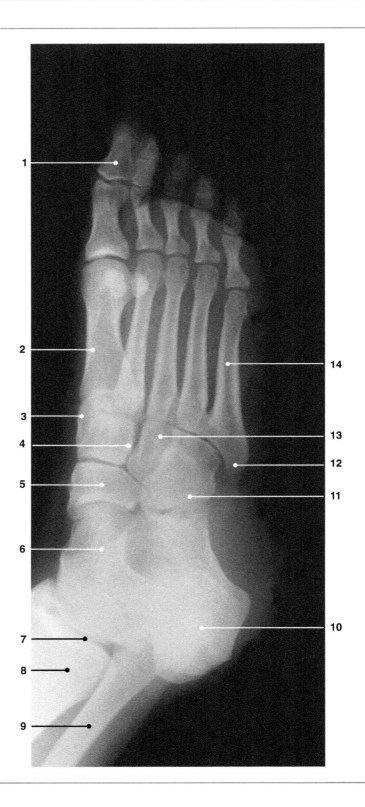

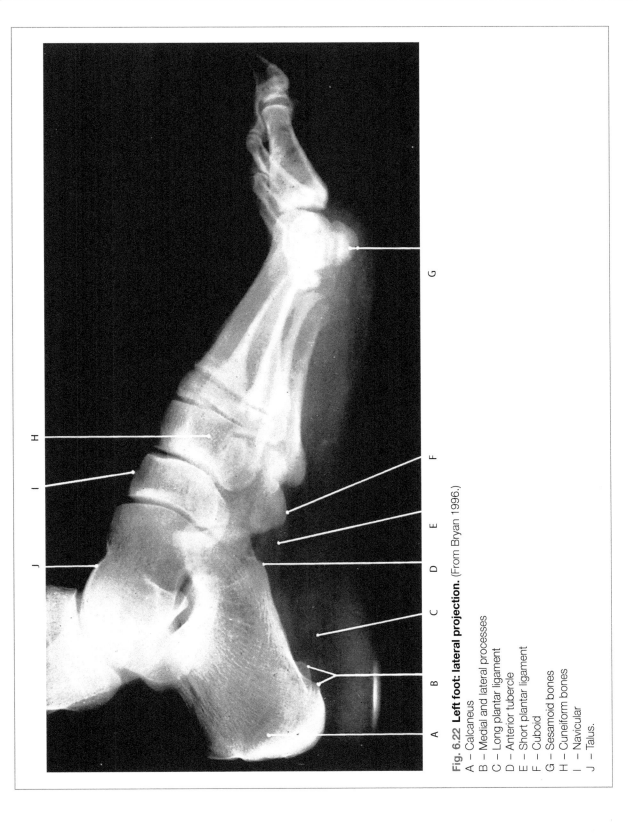

Fig. 6.22 Left foot: lateral projection. (From Bryan 1996.)

A – Calcaneus
B – Medial and lateral processes
C – Long plantar ligament
D – Anterior tubercle
E – Short plantar ligament
F – Cuboid
G – Sesamoid bones
H – Cuneiform bones
I – Navicular
J – Talus.

Fractures

Calcaneus

Cause – compression, due to a fall from a height onto both heels.

Example of treatment – bed rest for 4–6 weeks; physiotherapy. Arthrodesis if pain persists.

Metatarsals

Cause – direct blow, often due to a heavy object falling on the foot.

Example of treatment – walking plaster (below knee) for 3–4 weeks.

March fracture

Shafts of the metatarsals.

Cause – prolonged walking.

Example of treatment – often no treatment required. If severe pain, walking plaster (below knee) for 3–4 weeks.

Phalanges

Cause – crush injury.

Example of treatment – soft dressing.

Pathology

Gout (Fig. 6.23)

Disorder of protein metabolism with uric acid crystals deposited into the joints. Great toe is the most common site. Joints become swollen, red and painful.

Radiological signs – erosion of bone surfaces and soft tissue swelling.

Fig. 6.23 Gout. Radionuclide imaging. Note: Patient had normal radiographs. (From Resnick Kransdorf, 2005.)

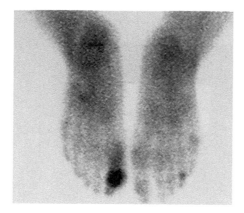

Hallux valgus (Fig. 6.24)

Lateral deviation of the great toe from the 1st metatarsal.

Cause – wearing tight fitting shoes.

Radiological sign – prominent 1st metatarsophalangeal joint is seen.

Pes planus (Fig. 6.25)

Flat feet.

Cause – muscular weakness (lack of muscle support stretches the ligaments).

Radiological sign – longitudinal arch of the foot is decreased.

Fig. 6.24 **Hallux valgus.** (Courtesy of Ernest Higginbottom.)

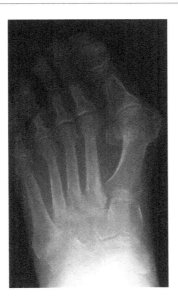

Fig. 6.25 **Pes planus.** (Courtesy of Ernest Higginbottom.)

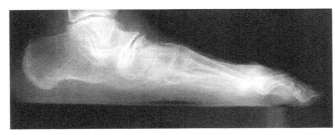

KNEE JOINT (Figs 6.26, 6.27, 6.28 and 6.29)

Type	Synovial condylar joint.

INSIGHT

In some publications the knee joint is incorrectly classified as a hinge joint. This is incorrect as when the joint is flexed there is a slight amount of medial and lateral rotation making it a synovial condylar joint.

Bony articular surfaces	The femoral condyles with the tibial condyles. Posterior aspect of the patella with the patellar articular surface of the femur. The articular surfaces are covered with articular hyaline cartilage.
Fibrous capsule	Blends with the suprapatellar tendon and the patellar ligament; elsewhere it is attached to the margins of the femoral and tibial condyles and to the head of the fibula.

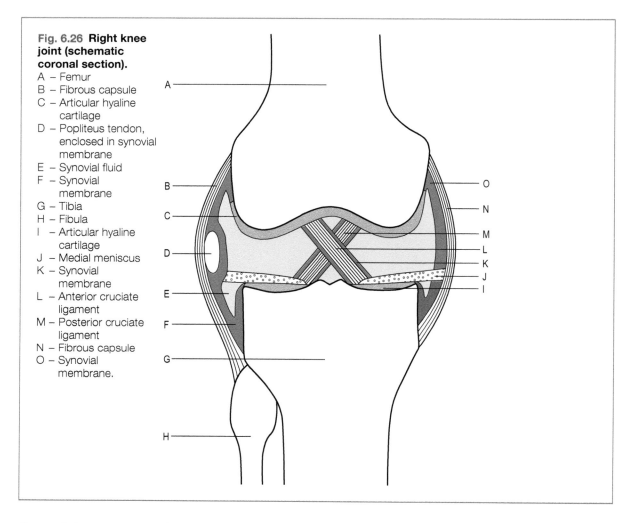

Fig. 6.26 Right knee joint (schematic coronal section).
A – Femur
B – Fibrous capsule
C – Articular hyaline cartilage
D – Popliteus tendon, enclosed in synovial membrane
E – Synovial fluid
F – Synovial membrane
G – Tibia
H – Fibula
I – Articular hyaline cartilage
J – Medial meniscus
K – Synovial membrane
L – Anterior cruciate ligament
M – Posterior cruciate ligament
N – Fibrous capsule
O – Synovial membrane.

Synovial membrane

Lines part of the fibrous capsule, and covers the intracapsular popliteus tendon. Anteriorly it forms the suprapatellar bursa and covers the anterior and lateral surfaces of the cruciate ligaments. The central posterior aspect of the joint has no synovial covering. The membrane secretes synovial fluid, which lubricates the joint.

Suprapatellar bursa – a sac containing synovial fluid, situated above the patella between the lower end of femur and the suprapatellar tendon.

Prepatellar bursa – a sac containing synovial fluid, situated between the anterior surface of the patella and the skin.

Infrapatellar bursa – a sac containing synovial fluid, situated below the patella between the upper tibia and the patellar ligament.

Supporting ligaments and tendons

Quadriceps femoris – attached to the superior aspect of the patella by the suprapatellar tendon.

Patellar ligament – attached to the inferior aspect of the patella and inserted into the tibial tuberosity.

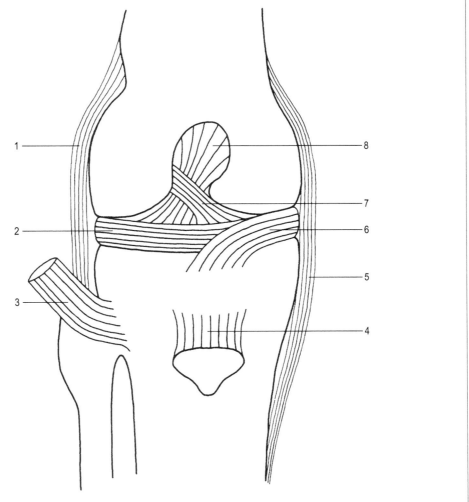

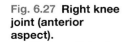

Fig. 6.27 Right knee joint (anterior aspect).
1 – Fibular collateral ligament
2 – Lateral meniscus
3 – Iliotibial tract
4 – Patellar ligament
5 – Tibial collateral ligament
6 – Medial meniscus
7 – Anterior cruciate ligament
8 – Posterior cruciate ligament.

Oblique popliteal – lateral aspect of the joint; blends with the fibrous capsule. The semimembranosus expands to form the oblique popliteal and is attached to the lateral condyle of the femur.

Arcuate popliteal – Y-shaped ligament on the lateral aspect of the joint, from the head of the fibula and the lateral epicondyle of the femur, arching over the popliteus tendon.

Tibial collateral – attached to the medial condyle of the tibia and the medial epicondyle of the femur.

Fibular collateral – lateral epicondyle of the femur to the head of the fibula.

Intracapsular structure

Anterior cruciate – medial part of the intercondylar area of the tibia to the medial surface of the lateral condyle of the femur.

Posterior cruciate – posterior part of the intercondylar area of the tibia to the lateral surface of the medial condyle of the femur.

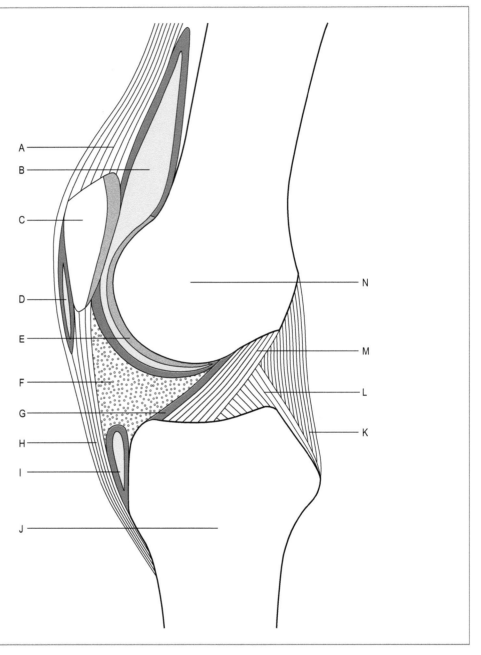

Fig. 6.28 Left knee joint (sagittal section).

A – Suprapatellar tendon
B – Suprapatellar bursa
C – Patella
D – Subcutaneous prepatellar bursa
E – Articular hyaline cartilage
F – Intrapatellar pad of fat
G – Synovial membrane
H – Patellar ligament
I – Deep intrapatellar bursa
J – Tibia
K – Fibrous capsule
L – Posterior cruciate ligament
M – Anterior cruciate ligament
N – Femur.

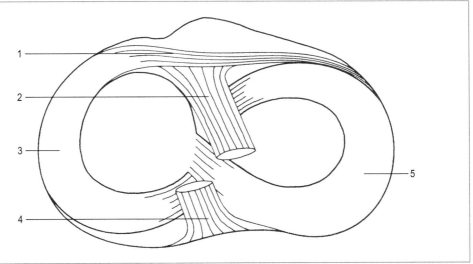

Fig. 6.29 Right tibia (superior aspect).
1 – Transverse ligament
2 – Anterior cruciate ligament
3 – Medial meniscus
4 – Posterior cruciate ligament
5 – Lateral meniscus.

Medial semilunar cartilage (meniscus) – situated on the medial aspect of the upper end of the tibia. The peripheral border is attached to the fibrous capsule.

Lateral semilunar cartilage (meniscus) – situated on the lateral aspect of the upper end of the tibia.

Infrapatellar pad of fat – situated above the infrapatellar bursa between the patellar ligament and the synovial membrane.

Movements

Flexion by the hamstring muscles aided by the gastrocnemius.
Extension by the quadriceps femoris.
When the knee is in flexion there is a minimal degree of:
Medial rotation by the popliteus.
Lateral rotation by the biceps femoris.

Blood supply

Branches of the femoral, popliteal and anterior tibial arteries, forming an anastomosis.

Nerve supply

Obturator, femoral, tibial and common peroneal nerves.

Fabella

Sesamoid bone found in the lateral head of gastrocnemius muscle where it passes over the lateral condyle of the femur. Smooth, round structure posterior to the knee joint on a lateral radiograph.

Radiographic appearances of the knee (Figs 6.30 to 6.35)

Fig. 6.30 Left knee: anteroposterior projection. (From Bryan 1996.)

A – Adductor tubercle
B – Medial epicondyle
C – Medial condyle
D – Tubercles of intercondylar eminence
E – Medial condyle
F – Tibia
G – Fibula
H – Lateral condyle
I – Lateral condyle
J – Lateral epicondyle
K – Patella
L – Femur.

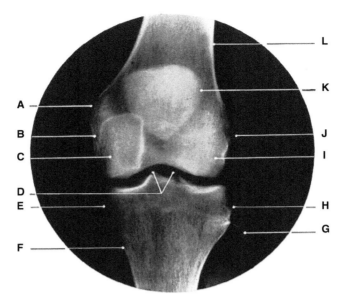

Fig. 6.31 Left knee: lateral projection. (From Bryan 1996.)

1 – Femur
2 – Intercondylar notch
3 – Condyles of femur
4 – Intercondylar eminence
5 – Superior tibiofibular joint
6 – Fibula
7 – Tibia
8 – Tibial tuberosity
9 – Ligamentum patellae
10 – Apex
11 – Patella
12 – Quadriceps femoris.

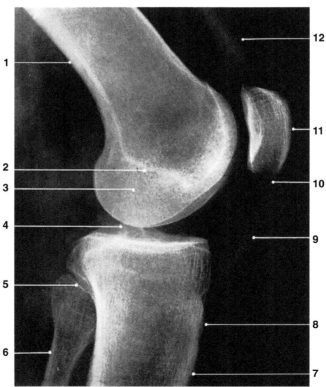

Fig. 6.32 Left knee: CT scan. (From Bryan 1996.)
A – Fabella
B – Femur
C – Patella.

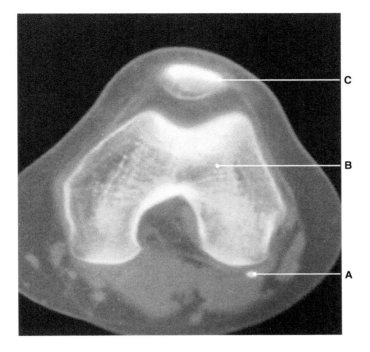

Fig. 6.33 Knee: MR scan. (From Bryan 1996.)
1 – Patella
2 – Patellar tendon
3 – Tibia
4 – Popliteal vessel
5 – Shaft of femur.

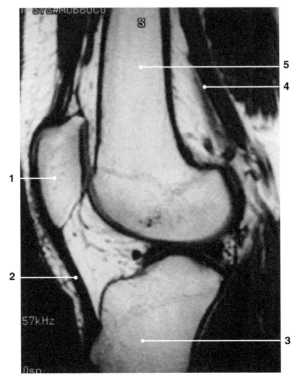

Fig. 6.34 **Normal lateral meniscus of the knee (arrowed). MR scan.**
(From Resnick Kransdorf, 2005.)

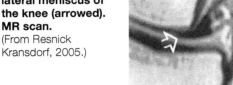

Fig. 6.35 **Normal collateral ligaments of the knee (arrowed). Ultrasound scan.**
(From Resnick Kransdorf, 2005.)
F – medial femoral condyle,
T – medial tibial plateau.

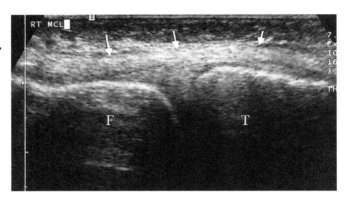

Pathology

Osteochondritis dissecans	*Cause* – local bone necrosis resulting in loose fragments of bone in the joint space.
	Radiological signs – dense bone fragments in the region of the femoral condyle, loose bodies within the joint capsule.
Osgood–Schlatter's disease (see Fig. 3.18)	Non-inflammatory condition affecting the tibial tuberosity.
	Cause – unknown. May be due to defective blood supply causing necrosis. It is an example of juvenile osteochondritis.
	Radiological signs – increased bone density and fragmentation of the area.
Torn meniscus (Fig. 6.36)	*Cause* – usually a twisting force, e.g. football injury. The medial meniscus is torn more commonly than the lateral.
	Radiological signs – demonstrated by arthrography (the radiographic examination of the intracapsular structures of the joint following the direct injection of a contrast agent into the joint cavity).

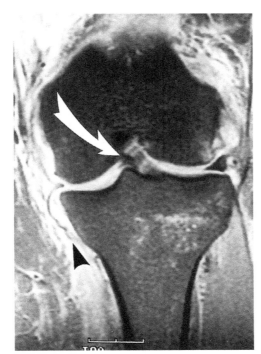

Fig. 6.36 **Medial collateral ligament tear (arrowhead) and displaced medial meniscus (arrowed). MR scan.** (From Resnick Kransdorf, 2005.)

SUPERIOR TIBIOFIBULAR JOINT

Type	Synovial plane joint.
Bony articular surfaces	Lateral condyle of the tibia with the head of fibula. Both surfaces are covered with articular hyaline cartilage.
Fibrous capsule	Attached to the margins of the articular facets on the tibia and fibula.
Synovial membrane	Lines the fibrous capsule and secretes synovial fluid, which lubricates the joint.
Supporting ligaments	Anterior ligament.
Movements	Gliding.
Blood supply	Branches of the anterior tibial artery.
Nerve supply	Common peroneal nerve.

Radiographic appearances of the superior tibiofibular joint (Fig. 6.37)

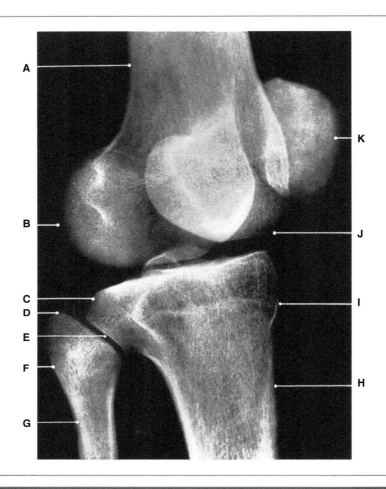

Fig. 6.37 Left superior tibiofibular joint: oblique projection. (From Bryan 1996.)
A – Femur
B – Lateral condyle
C – Lateral condyle
D – Styloid process
E – Superior tibiofibular joint
F – Head
G – Fibula
H – Tibia
I – Medial condyle
J – Medial condyle
K – Patella.

INFERIOR TIBIOFIBULAR JOINT

Type	Fibrous syndesmoses.
Bony articular surfaces	Lower end of fibula and the fibular notch of the tibia.
Strengthening ligaments	*Anterior tibiofibular ligament.* *Posterior tibiofibular ligament.* *Interosseous ligament.*
Movements	Minimal.
Blood supply	Branches of the peroneal artery; branches of the anterior and posterior tibial arteries.
Nerve supply	Deep peroneal, tibial and saphenous nerves.

ANKLE JOINT (Figs 6.38 and 6.39)

Type

Synovial saddle joint (*not* a synovial hinge joint due to the accessory movements in plantar-flexion).

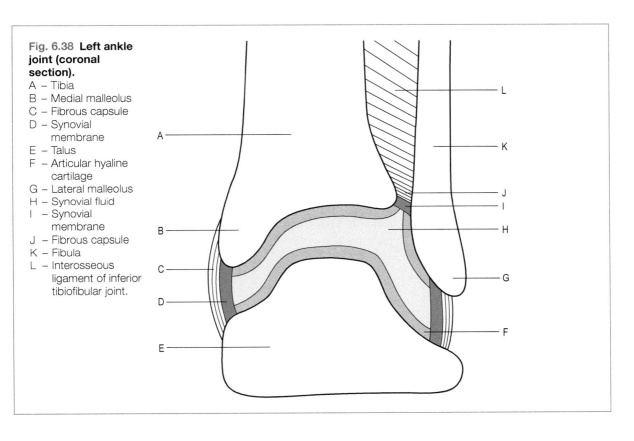

Fig. 6.38 Left ankle joint (coronal section).
A – Tibia
B – Medial malleolus
C – Fibrous capsule
D – Synovial membrane
E – Talus
F – Articular hyaline cartilage
G – Lateral malleolus
H – Synovial fluid
I – Synovial membrane
J – Fibrous capsule
K – Fibula
L – Interosseous ligament of inferior tibiofibular joint.

Bony articular surfaces

The distal end and the medial malleolus of the tibia, the medial aspect of the lateral malleolus of the fibula, with the talus. The articular surfaces are covered with articular hyaline cartilage.

Fibrous capsule

Attached to the tibia and fibula above the malleoli; to the posterior and lateral surfaces of the talus and anteriorly to the neck of the talus. The capsule is weak anteriorly and posteriorly but is strengthened laterally by ligaments.

Synovial membrane

Lines the fibrous capsule and the parts of the bone not covered with articular hyaline cartilage. A small fold extends between the distal ends of the tibia and fibula. The synovial membrane secretes synovial fluid, which lubricates the joint.

Supporting ligaments

Medial collateral or deltoid – apex attached to the medial malleolus, and the base to the navicular, calcaneus and talus.

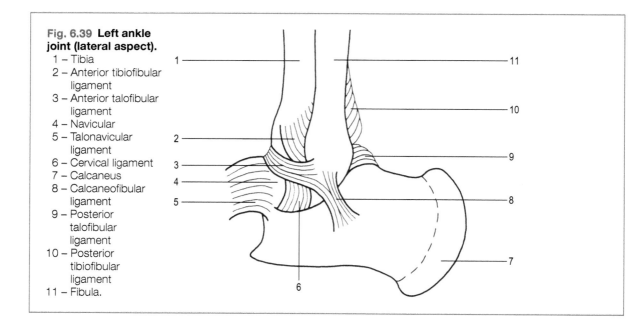

Fig. 6.39 Left ankle joint (lateral aspect).
1 – Tibia
2 – Anterior tibiofibular ligament
3 – Anterior talofibular ligament
4 – Navicular
5 – Talonavicular ligament
6 – Cervical ligament
7 – Calcaneus
8 – Calcaneofibular ligament
9 – Posterior talofibular ligament
10 – Posterior tibiofibular ligament
11 – Fibula.

Lateral collateral – consists of 3 ligaments:
Anterior talofibular – attached to the lateral malleolus and the talus
Posterior talofibular – attached to the malleolar fossa and the talus
Calcaneofibular – attached to the lateral malleolus and the calcaneus.

Movements

Main movements
Dorsiflexion by the anterior tibialis muscle.
Plantarflexion by the soleus and gastrocnemius.

Accessory movements
Abduction
Adduction } slight movement in plantar-flexion.
Rotation

Blood supply   Branches of the anterior tibial and peroneal arteries.

Nerve supply   Posterior and lateral popliteal nerves.

Radiographic appearances of the ankle joint (Figs 6.40, 6.41, 6.42 and 6.43)

Fig. 6.40 **Left ankle joint: anteroposterior projection.** (From Bryan 1996.)
A – Tibia
B – Medial malleolus
C – Trochlear surface of talus
D – Malleolar fossa
E – Lateral malleolus
F – Inferior tibiofibular joint
G – Fibula.

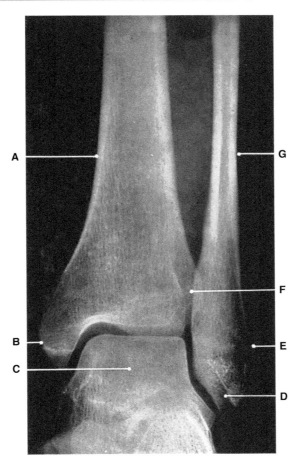

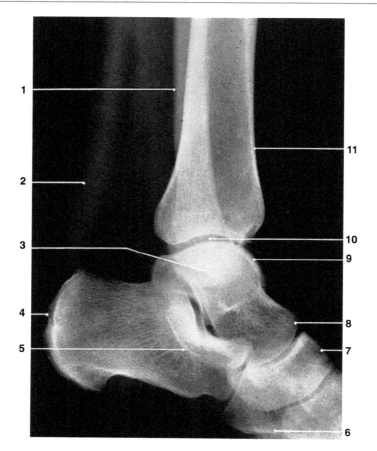

Fig. 6.41 Left ankle joint: lateral projection.
(From Bryan 1996.)
1 – Fibula
2 – Tendo calcaneus
3 – Malleoli medial and lateral
4 – Calcaneus
5 – Sustentaculum tali
6 – Cuboid
7 – Navicular
8 – Head of talus
9 – Trochlear surface of talus
10 – Ankle joint
11 – Tibia.

Fig. 6.42 Ankle joint: MR scan, sagittal section. (From Bryan 1996.)

A – Ankle joint
B – Talus
C – Navicular
D – Calcaneus
E – Posterior talo-
      calcaneal joint
F – Achilles tendon
G – Tibia.

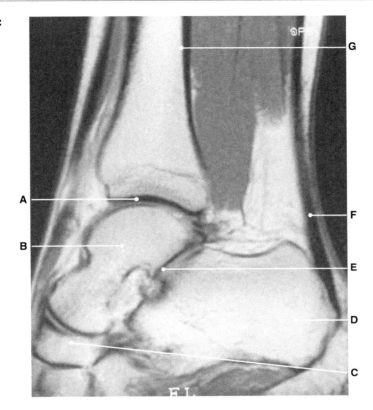

Fig. 6.43 Normal anterior fibular ligament (curved arrow) and posterior talofibular ligament (open arrow). MR scan. (From Resnick Kransdorf, 2005.)

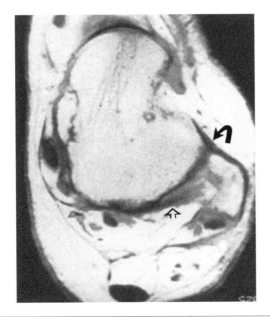

Fractures

INSIGHT

A fracture of the lower end of the tibia has often an associated fracture of the neck of fibula, therefore it is important to image the knee joint if a fracture is seen.

Pott's fracture
(Fig. 6.44)

Cause – external rotation of the foot.

First degree
Oblique fracture of lower end of tibia with no displacement.

Example of treatment – plaster of Paris, below knee walking plaster.

Second degree
Oblique fracture of lower end of fibula, transverse fracture of medial malleolus.

Example of treatment – open or closed reduction; screws may be inserted. Plaster of Paris, below knee walking plaster.

Third degree
As second degree but with vertical fracture of the lower end of the tibia.

Example of treatment – see Second degree.

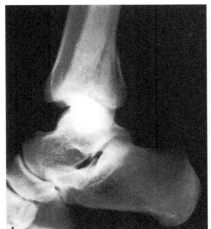
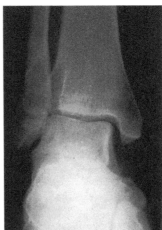
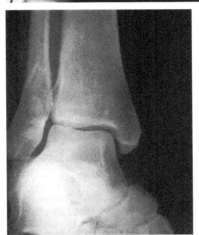

Fig. 6.44 **Pott's fracture (first degree).** (From Sutton 1987.)

Pathology

Torn lateral ligament

Cause – internal rotation of the foot.

Example of treatment – adhesive strapping or plaster of Paris, below knee walking plaster.

Radiological signs – joint space is widened laterally, demonstrated by an antero-posterior radiograph of the ankle joint with forced inversion.

Torn Achilles tendon (Fig 6.45)

Cause – Violent stretching of the tendon.

Example of treatment – surgical repair may be required.

Fig 6.45 Torn Achilles tendon. MR scan. (From Resnick Kransdorf, 2005.)

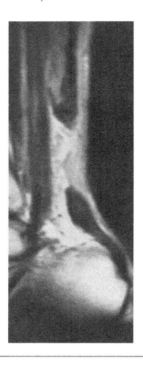

Pelvic girdle

CHAPTER CONTENTS

The pelvic girdle is formed by the 2 hip bones, the sacrum and the coccyx. For notes on the sacrum and coccyx, see Chapter 9.

HIP BONE (Figs 7.1 and 7.2)

This is a large, irregularly shaped bone composed of 3 bones – the ilium, ischium and pubis – which are fused together in the adult.

Ilium (Figs 7.1 and 7.2)

Type	Flat bone
Position	Forms the superior aspect of the hip bone, lying mainly above the acetabulum.
Articulations	*The auricular surface of the ilium* with the auricular facet of the sacrum to form the sacroiliac joint. *The ilium forms part of the acetabulum,* which articulates with the head of the femur to form the hip joint.
Main parts	*Iliac crest* – forms the superior border, which is easily palpated and provides attachment for numerous abdominal muscles. The highest part of the crest lies at the level of the 4th lumbar vertebra. *Anterior superior iliac spine* – easily palpated and lies at the lateral end of the iliac crest. *Anterior inferior iliac spine* – a bony prominence immediately above the acetabulum. *Anterior border* – from the anterior superior iliac spine to the acetabulum. *Posterior superior iliac spine* – lies at the posterior border of the iliac crest.

Fig. 7.1 Hip bone (external aspect).

Ilium
A – Iliac crest
B – Anterior superior iliac spine
C – Inferior gluteal line
D – Anterior inferior iliac spine
E – Acetabulum
F – Greater sciatic notch
G – Posterior inferior iliac spine
H – Posterior superior iliac spine.

Pubis
1 – Superior ramus
2 – Pubic tubercle
3 – Obturator foramen
4 – Inferior ramus.

Ischium
a – Ischial ramus
b – Ischial tuberosity
c – Lesser sciatic notch
d – Ischial spine.

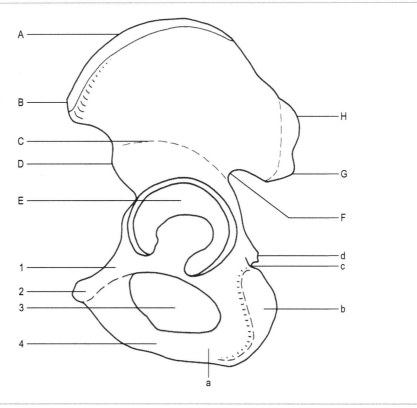

Posterior inferior iliac spine – lies approximately 2.5 cm below the posterior superior iliac spine.

Posterior border – curved border from the posterior superior iliac spine to the posterior border of the ischium.

Greater sciatic notch – lies below the posterior inferior iliac spine. The sciatic nerve leaves the pelvis via the notch.

Internal (medial) surface – divided into 2 areas, the iliac fossa and the sacro-pelvic surface, which are separated by the medial border.

Iliac fossa – concave surface for the iliacus muscle.

Sacropelvic surface – situated between the medial and posterior borders, and divided into 3 areas:

    Iliac tuberosity – upper part, roughened for ligament attachment.
    Auricular surface – middle part, for articulation with the sacrum.
    Pelvic surface – lower part, forms part of the wall of the true pelvis.

Medial border – forms part of the arcuate line (the border between the 'true' and 'false' pelvis).

External (lateral) surface – consists of a large gluteal surface superiorly and a small area inferiorly which forms part of the acetabulum.

Fig. 7.2 Hip bone (internal aspect).

Ilium
I – Iliac crest
J – Posterior superior iliac spine
K – Auricular surface
L – Posterior inferior iliac spine
M – Greater sciatic notch
N – Iliopubic eminence
O – Medial border
P – Anterior superior iliac spine
Q – Iliac fossa.

Pubis
5 – Inferior ramus
6 – Obturator foramen
7 – Articular area for symphysis pubis
8 – Pubic tubercle
9 – Superior ramus.

Ischium
e – Ischial spine
f – Lesser sciatic notch
g – Body
h – Ischial tuberosity
i – Ischial ramus

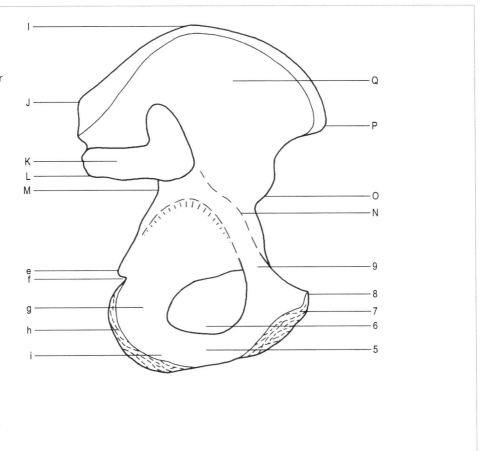

Gluteal surface – crossed by 3 roughened ridges for attachment of the gluteal muscles.

Iliopubic eminence – at the junction of the ilium and the pubis. Lies at the anterior aspect of the medial border.

Ischium (Figs 7.1 and 7.2)

Type	Flat bone.
Position	Forms the posterior and inferior portion of the hip bone.
Articulations	*The ischium forms part of the acetabulum,* which articulates with the head of femur to form the hip joint.
Main parts	*Body* – forms part of the acetabulum and the greater sciatic notch.
	Ischial tuberosity – roughened area on the posterior and inferior aspect of the body; forms attachment for the hamstrings, long head of biceps femoris and semimembranosus.

Ischial spine – at the lower end of the greater sciatic notch, for the sacrospinous ligament.

Lesser sciatic notch – below the ischial spine.

Ischial ramus – thin portion of bone on the inferior aspect; is continuous with the pubic ramus.

Pubis (Figs 7.1 and 7.2)

Type

Flat bone.

Position

Forms the inferior and medial aspect of the hip bone.

Articulations

The pubis forms part of the acetabulum, which articulates with the head of the femur to form the hip joint.
The right and left pubic bones articulate with each other to form the symphysis pubis.

Main parts

Body – forms the anterior wall of the true pelvis and articulates with the opposite pubic bone to form the symphysis pubis.

Pubic crest – subcutaneous and forms the upper border of the body.

Pubic tubercle – on the lateral aspect of the pubic crest, for the inguinal ligament.

Superior ramus – forms part of the acetabulum.

Inferior ramus – extends downwards and laterally to join the ramus of the ischium.

Obturator foramen – large opening formed by the ischium (body and ramus) and the pubis (superior and inferior rami). The foramen is occupied by the obturator membrane.

Acetabulum (Fig. 7.3)
Cup-shaped socket on the lateral aspect of the hip bone for articulation with the head of the femur. Formed by the pubis (anterior fifth), ischium (posterior two-fifths) and ilium (superior two-fifths).

Acetabular notch – deficiency in the inferior aspect of the acetabular rim.

Acetabular fossa – forms the base of the acetabulum and is non-articular.

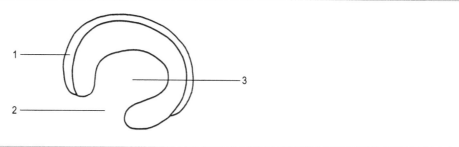

Fig. 7.3 Acetabulum.
1 – Acetabular rim
2 – Acetabular notch
3 – Acetabular fossa.

Ossification

Primary centres

Ilium – 8th week intrauterine life.

Ischium – age 4 months.

Pubis – age 4–5 months.

Secondary centres

Ilium – 2 centres:

iliac crest appears at puberty;

anterior inferior iliac spine appears at puberty.

Ischium – 1 centre:

ischial tuberosity appears at puberty.

Pubis – 1 centre:

symphysis pubis appears at puberty.

The hip bone fuses age 15–25.

THE PELVIS (Figs 7.4 and 7.5)

The pelvis is formed posteriorly by the sacrum and coccyx and anteriorly by the two hip bones.

The greater (false) pelvis

The upper portion of the pelvis is referred to as the greater pelvis. It is larger than the lesser (true) pelvis and lies *above the pelvic brim*; the pelvic brim is the oblique plane formed by the sacral promontory posteriorly, the arcuate line of the ilium and the pecten pubis (iliopectineal line) laterally and the pubic tubercle and crest and the upper border of the symphysis pubis anteriorly. The greater pelvis forms part of the abdominal cavity.

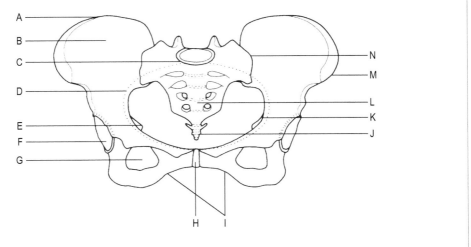

Fig. 7.4 Female pelvis (anterior aspect).

A – Iliac crest

B – Iliac fossa

C – Sacral promontory

D – Arcuate line

E – Ischial spine

F – Acetabulum

G – Obturator foramen

H – Symphysis pubis

I – Pubic arch

J – Coccyx

K – Pelvic brim

L – Sacrum

M – Anterior superior iliac spine

N – Sacroiliac joint.

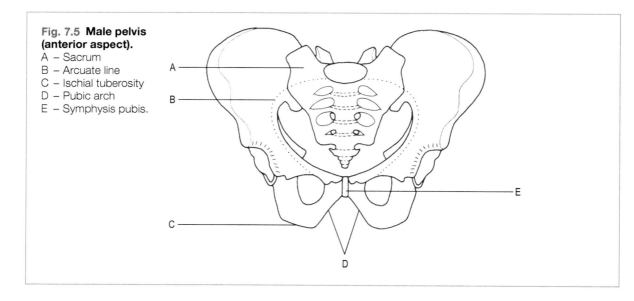

Fig. 7.5 Male pelvis (anterior aspect).
A – Sacrum
B – Arcuate line
C – Ischial tuberosity
D – Pubic arch
E – Symphysis pubis.

The lesser (true) pelvis

The lesser pelvis lies *below the pelvic brim* and can be divided into 3 areas:

The pelvic inlet
Bounded by the pelvic brim.
 Male – heart-shaped.
 Female – circular.

The pelvic outlet
Formed by the *pubic arch* – the rami of the ischium and pubis anteriorly the sacrotuberous ligaments and the ischial tuberosities laterally and the apex of the sacrum posteriorly.

The pelvic cavity
The area between the inlet and the outlet contains the rectum, bladder and parts of the reproductive system.

Table 7.1 Differences between the male and female pelvis

	Male	**Female**
General shape	Narrow, deep	Wide, shallow
Bone structure	Heavy	Light
Pelvic cavity	Long, tapering downwards	Short, cylindrical
Sacrum	Narrow, long, curved	Wide, short, less curved
Pelvic inlet	Heart-shaped	Circular
Ischial tuberosities	Close	Wide apart
Pubic arch	Less than 90°	More than 90°
Greater sciatic notch	Acute, narrow	90°, wide
Symphysis pubis	Limited movement	More flexible

Radiographic appearances of the pelvis (Figs 7.6 and 7.7)

Fig. 7.6 Male pelvis: anteroposterior projection.
(From Bryan 1996.)
A – Gas-filled caecum
B – Anterior superior iliac spine
C – Brim of pelvis
D – Acetabulum
E – Obturator foramen
F – Pubic arch
G – Ischial tuberosity
H – Fovea of femur
I – Anterior inferior iliac spine
J – Sacroiliac joint
K – Iliac fossa
L – Iliac crest
M – 5th lumbar vertebra.

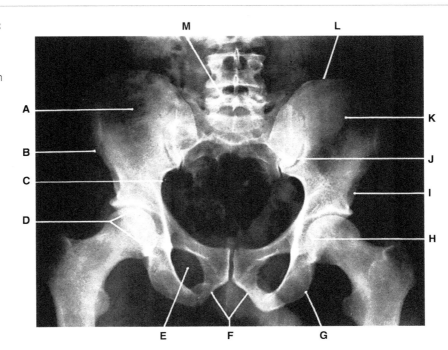

Fig. 7.7 Female pelvis: anteroposterior projection.
(From Bryan 1996.)
1 – Sacrum
2 – Greater trochanter
3 – Coccyx
4 – Symphysis pubis
5 – Pubic arch
6 – Head of femur
7 – Pelvic brim
8 – Posterior superior iliac spine.

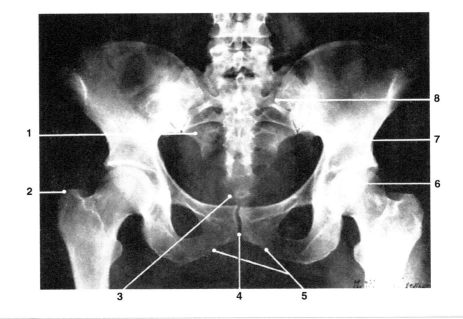

Measurement of pelvic size (Figs 7.8 and 7.9)

It is sometimes necessary to establish that the pelvis is of a suitable size to permit the normal passage of a fetus.

Measurement of the pelvic inlet

True conjugate diameter – the anteroposterior measurement from the upper, inner border of the symphysis pubis to the sacral promontory in the midline.

Transverse diameter – the maximum distance across the pubic inlet.

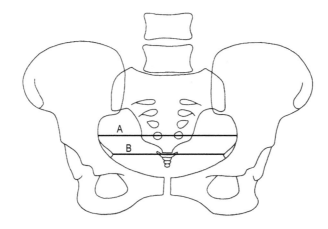

Fig. 7.8 Pelvic measurements (anterior aspect).
A – Transverse diameter
B – Interspinous diameter.

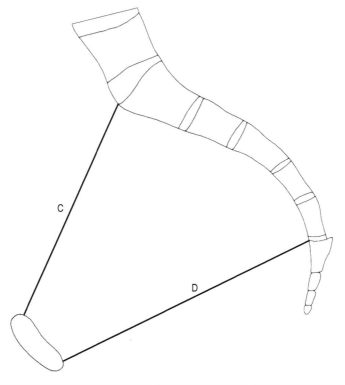

Fig. 7.9 Pelvic measurements (lateral aspect).
C – True conjugate diameter
D – Anteroposterior diameter.

Measurement of the pelvic outlet

Anteroposterior diameter – between the lower, inner border of the symphysis pubis and the apex of the sacrum.

Intertuberous diameter – between the ischial tuberosities.

Interspinous diameter – between the ischial spines.

Fractures

INSIGHT

A fracture of the pelvis always has either a second fracture or a dislocation of one of the joints. Think of a polo mint – it is impossible to break it in one place.

Isolated fracture of either the superior or inferior ischiopubic ramus, ilium or acetabulum

Cause – direct blow (may be the cause of damage to the bladder or urethra).

Example of treatment – bed rest 2–3 weeks.

Contrecoup fracture

Fractures which disrupt the pelvic ring.

Cause – severe blow, e.g. road traffic accidents (usually cause damage to the bladder, urethra, major blood vessels).

Example of treatment – bed rest.

HIP JOINT (Figs 7.10 and 7.11)

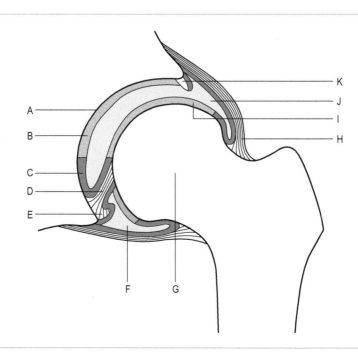

Fig. 7.10 Left hip joint (coronal section).

A – Acetabulum
B – Articular hyaline cartilage
C – Synovial membrane
D – Ligament of head of femur
E – Transverse acetabular ligament
F – Synovial fluid
G – Head of femur
H – Fibrous capsule
I – Articular hyaline cartilage
J – Synovial fluid
K – Acetabular labrum.

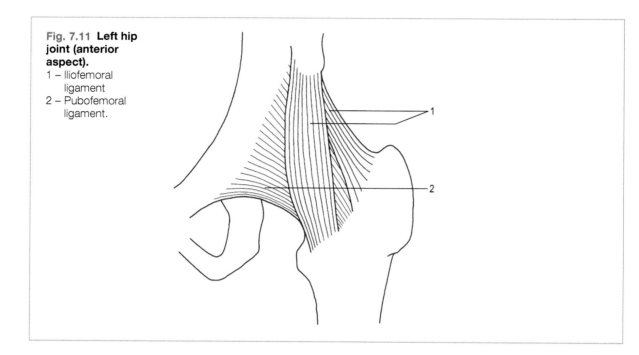

Fig. 7.11 Left hip joint (anterior aspect).
1 – Iliofemoral ligament
2 – Pubofemoral ligament.

Type	Synovial ball and socket joint.
Bony articular surfaces	The head of the femur with the acetabulum of the hip bone. The articular surfaces are covered with articular hyaline cartilage, except for the fovea of the head of femur.
Fibrous capsule	Attached medially to the edge of the acetabulum, the acetabular labrum and the transverse acetabular ligament, anteriorly to the intertrochanteric line and laterally to the neck of femur. The capsule is loose inferiorly to allow movement.
Synovial membrane	Lines the fibrous capsule and covers the ligament of the head of femur, the intracapsular part of the neck of femur and the pad of fat in the acetabular fossa. The membrane secretes synovial fluid, which lubricates the joint.
Supporting ligaments	*Iliofemoral ligament* – triangular-shaped and located anteriorly. The apex is attached to the anterior inferior iliac spine and the base to the intertrochanteric line of the femur.
	Ischiofemoral ligament – posteriorly, from the ischium to the intertrochanteric crest.
	Pubofemoral ligament – anteriorly, from the pubis to the intertrochanteric line. Its fibres blend with those of the fibrous capsule and the iliofemoral ligament.

Ligament of the head of femur – triangular-shaped. The apex is attached to the fovea of the head of femur and the base to the acetabular notch and the transverse ligament.

Transverse acetabular ligament – connects the inferior aspect of the acetabular labrum bridging the acetabular notch.

Intracapsular structures	*Acetabular labrum* – fibrocartilaginous rim round the acetabulum to deepen the socket. *Pad of fat* – lies in the acetabular fossa.
Movements	*Flexion* by the iliacus and the psoas assisted by the rectus femoris. *Extension* by the gluteus maximus, assisted by the hamstrings. *Abduction* by the gluteus medius and the gluteus minimus. *Adduction* by the adductor muscles. *Medial rotation* by the anterior parts of the gluteus medius, the gluteus minimus and the tensor fasciae latae. *Lateral rotation* by the obturator, gemelli and quadriceps femoris. *Circumduction* by a combination of the above movements.
Blood supply	Branches of the obturator, gluteal and femoral arteries.
Nerve supply	Branches of the femoral, obturator and gluteal nerves.

Radiographic appearances of the hip joint (Figs 7.12, 7.13 and 7.14)

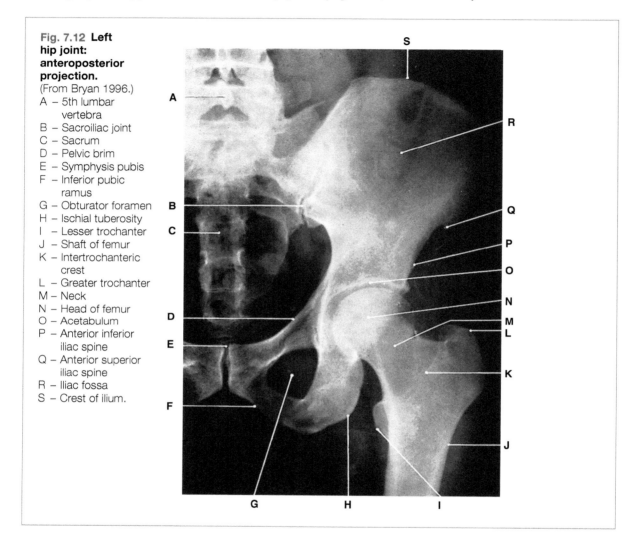

Fig. 7.12 Left hip joint: anteroposterior projection.
(From Bryan 1996.)
A – 5th lumbar vertebra
B – Sacroiliac joint
C – Sacrum
D – Pelvic brim
E – Symphysis pubis
F – Inferior pubic ramus
G – Obturator foramen
H – Ischial tuberosity
I – Lesser trochanter
J – Shaft of femur
K – Intertrochanteric crest
L – Greater trochanter
M – Neck
N – Head of femur
O – Acetabulum
P – Anterior inferior iliac spine
Q – Anterior superior iliac spine
R – Iliac fossa
S – Crest of ilium.

Fig. 7.13 Hip joint: lateral projection.
(From Bryan 1996.)
1 – Ischial spine
2 – Acetabulum
3 – Ischial tuberosity
4 – Greater trochanter
5 – Lesser trochanter
6 – Shaft of femur
7 – Greater trochanter
8 – Neck of femur
9 – Head of femur
10 – Iliac crest
11 – Pubic ramus
12 – Symphysis pubis.

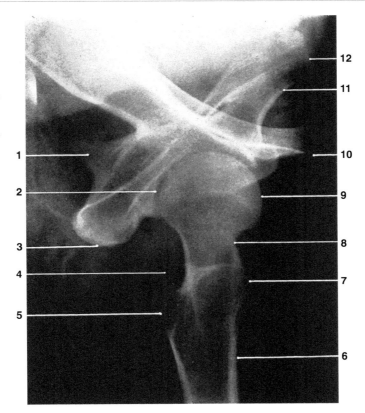

Fig. 7.14 Right hip joint: CT scan.
(From Bryan 1996.)
A – Greater trochanter
B – Acetabulum
C – Head of femur.

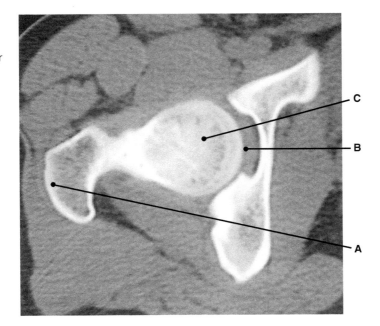

Trauma

Posterior dislocation and fracture dislocation

Cause – force driving the head of femur backwards out of the acetabulum, e.g. road traffic accident.

Example of treatment – reduction under anaesthetic. Traction for 4 weeks.

Anterior dislocation (rare)

Cause – forced abduction of the extended hip, e.g. road traffic accident.

Example of treatment – reduction under anaesthetic. Traction for 3 weeks.

Central fracture dislocation

Cause – heavy blow forcing the femoral head through the acetabulum. Example of treatment – traction.

Pathology

Congenital dislocation of the hip (Figs 7.15 and 7.16)

Shallow acetabulum – therefore the head of femur is displaced upwards.

Radiological signs – femoral head displaced upwards and outwards with delayed ossification of the epiphysis.

Fig. 7.15 **Congenital dislocation, right hip.** a. At age 1 year. b. Same patient at age 4 years 5 months. (Courtesy of Ernest Higginbottom.)

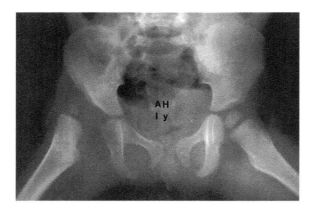

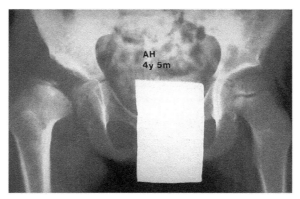

Fig. 7.16 Congenital dislocation, left hip, failed reduction. CT scan. (From Resnick Kransdorf, 2005.)

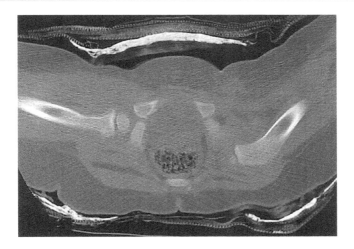

Slipped upper femoral epiphysis

Epiphysis is displaced backwards and downwards.
Radiological sign – imperfect alignment of the epiphysis with the neck of femur.

Perthes' disease (Fig. 7.17)

Osteochondritis of the epiphysis of the femoral head.
Radiological signs – widening of the epiphyseal line, irregular metaphyseal outline, flattened epiphysis. Some increase in bone density within the head of femur.

Fig. 7.17 Perthes' disease, *right femoral head.* (Courtesy of Ernest Higginbottom.)

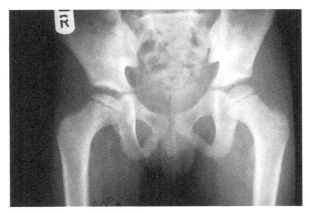

SACROILIAC JOINTS

Type

Synovial plane joint.

Bony articular surfaces

The articular surface of the ilium with the *auricular facet of the sacrum;* the joint spaces are directed obliquely forwards. The articular surface on the ilium is covered with articular hyaline cartilage and that on the sacrum with fibrocartilage.

Fibrous capsule

Attached medially to the sacrum and laterally to the ilium.

Synovial membrane

Lines the fibrous capsule. Secretes synovial fluid, which lubricates the joint.

Supporting ligaments

Ventral sacroiliac ligament – covers the anterior and inferior aspects of the joint.

Interosseous sacroiliac ligament – between the 2 bones; is very strong.

Dorsal sacroiliac ligament – covers the posterior aspect of the joint; merges with the sacrotuberous ligament.

Accessory ligaments
Sacrotuberous ligament.
Sacrospinous ligament.

Movements

Restricted to *slight anteroposterior rotation* during flexion and extension of the trunk.

Radiographic appearances of the sacroiliac joints (Figs 7.18, 7.19, 7.20 and 7.21)

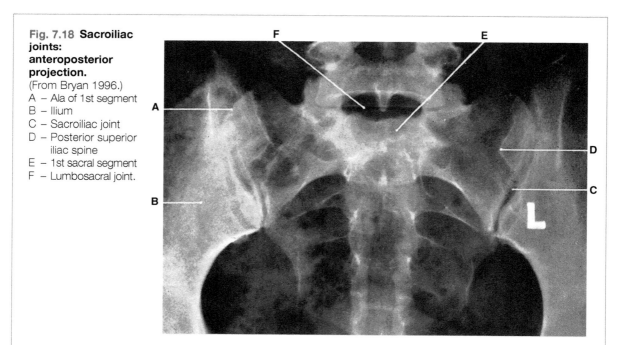

Fig. 7.18 Sacroiliac joints: anteroposterior projection.
(From Bryan 1996.)
A – Ala of 1st segment
B – Ilium
C – Sacroiliac joint
D – Posterior superior iliac spine
E – 1st sacral segment
F – Lumbosacral joint.

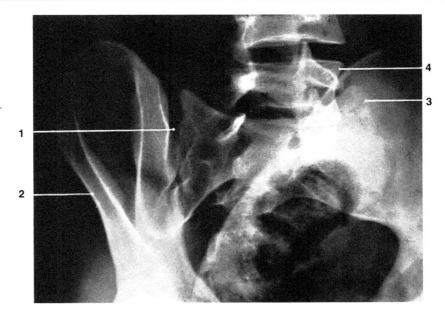

Fig. 7.19 Right sacroiliac joint: oblique projection.
(From Bryan 1996.)
1 – Sacroiliac joint
2 – Ilium
3 – Sacrum
4 – Body of 5th lumbar
   vertebra.

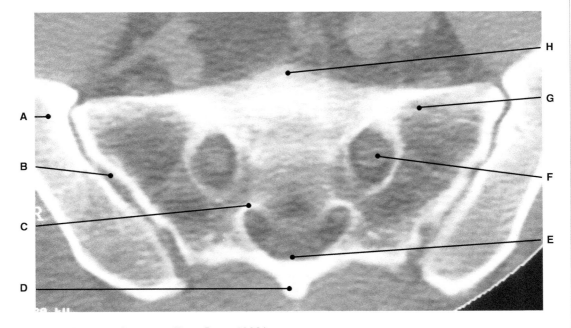

Fig. 7.20 Sacrum: CT scan. (From Bryan 1996.)
A – Ilium
B – Sacroiliac joint
C – Margin of sacral foramen
D – Spinous tubercle
E – Sacral canal
F – Anterior sacral foramen
G – Lateral mass of sacrum
H – Sacral promontory.

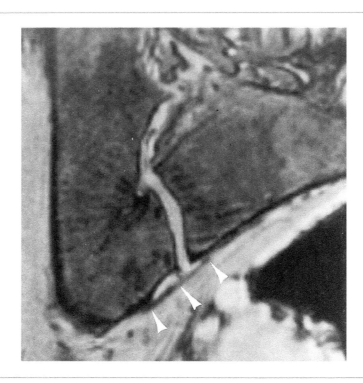

Fig. 7.21 **Ventral sacroiliac ligament (arrowed). MR scan.** (From Resnick Kransdorf, 2005.)

Pathology

Subluxation may occur.

SYMPHYSIS PUBIS

Type	Cartilaginous symphysis.
Bony articular surfaces	Right pubic body with left pubic body. The articular surfaces are covered with articular hyaline cartilage.
Supporting ligaments	*Superior pubic ligament* – covers the superior aspect. *Arcuate pubic ligament* – covers the inferior aspect.
Intracapsular structures	*Interpubic disc of fibrocartilage* – connects the 2 bones.
Movements	Minimal movement present.

Thorax

CHAPTER CONTENTS

STERNUM (Figs 8.1 and 8.2)

Type

Flat bone.

Position

Lies on the anterior aspect of the thorax in the midline.

Articulations

The clavicular notch with the sternal end of the clavicle to form the sternoclavicular joint.

Notches on the lateral aspect of the sternum articulate with the first 7 costal cartilages to form the sternocostal joints.

Main parts

Manubrium sterni

Jugular (suprasternal) notch on the superior border; lies at the level of the 2nd–3rd thoracic vertebrae.

Clavicular notches on either side of the jugular notch; articulate with the clavicles to form the sternoclavicular joints.

Facet for the 1st costal cartilage, at the upper end of the lateral border.

Demi-facet for the 2nd costal cartilage, at the lower end of the lateral border.

Inferior border articulates with the body to form the sternal angle, which lies at the level of the 4th–5th thoracic vertebrae and can be easily palpated.

Body

4 segments – form the long, thin body.

3 ridges – connect the segments.

4 notches – on each lateral aspect for the 3rd–6th costal cartilages.

2 demi-facets – on each lateral aspect for the 2nd and 7th costal cartilages.

Xiphoid process

Superior angle – completes the notch for the 7th costal cartilage.

Xiphisternal joint – at the junction of the body and the xiphoid process at the level of the 9th–10th thoracic vertebrae.

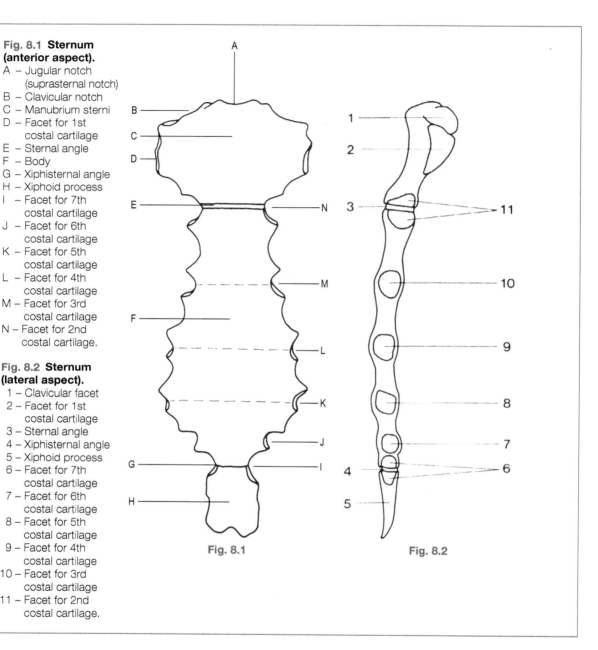

Fig. 8.1 Sternum (anterior aspect).
A – Jugular notch (suprasternal notch)
B – Clavicular notch
C – Manubrium sterni
D – Facet for 1st costal cartilage
E – Sternal angle
F – Body
G – Xiphisternal angle
H – Xiphoid process
I – Facet for 7th costal cartilage
J – Facet for 6th costal cartilage
K – Facet for 5th costal cartilage
L – Facet for 4th costal cartilage
M – Facet for 3rd costal cartilage
N – Facet for 2nd costal cartilage.

Fig. 8.2 Sternum (lateral aspect).
1 – Clavicular facet
2 – Facet for 1st costal cartilage
3 – Sternal angle
4 – Xiphisternal angle
5 – Xiphoid process
6 – Facet for 7th costal cartilage
7 – Facet for 6th costal cartilage
8 – Facet for 5th costal cartilage
9 – Facet for 4th costal cartilage
10 – Facet for 3rd costal cartilage
11 – Facet for 2nd costal cartilage.

Fig. 8.1

Fig. 8.2

Ossification

Primary centres

6 centres:

Manubrium – 5th month intrauterine life.

Body – 4 centres (1 per segment):
   1st and 2nd segments – 5th month of intrauterine life.
   3rd and 4th segments – 5th–6th month of intrauterine life.

Xiphoid process – age 3.

Body begins to fuse after puberty – from the inferior aspect to the superior aspect and continues to age 25.

Radiographic appearances of the sternum (Figs 8.3 and 8.4)

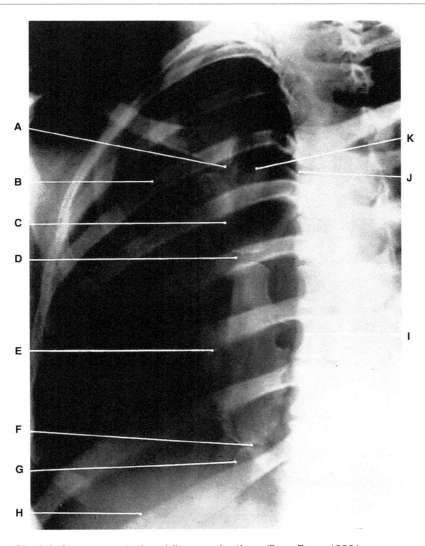

Fig. 8.3 **Sternum: anterior oblique projection.** (From Bryan 1996.)

A – Right sternoclavicular joint
B – 5th rib
C – Manubrium
D – Sternal angle
E – Body of sternum
F – Xiphisternal joint
G – Xiphoid process
H – 10th rib
I – Thoracic vertebra
J – Left sternoclavicular joint
K – Suprasternal notch.

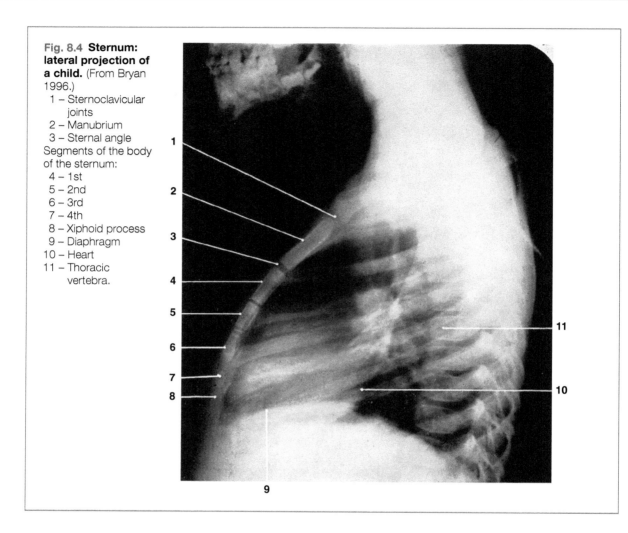

Fig. 8.4 Sternum: lateral projection of a child. (From Bryan 1996.)
1 – Sternoclavicular joints
2 – Manubrium
3 – Sternal angle
Segments of the body of the sternum:
4 – 1st
5 – 2nd
6 – 3rd
7 – 4th
8 – Xiphoid process
9 – Diaphragm
10 – Heart
11 – Thoracic vertebra.

Fractures

Depression of the body	With impaired respiration.
	Cause – direct blow.
	Example of treatment – may require elevation of the sternum.
Junction of the manubrium and the body	With associated fracture of the thoracic spine.
	Cause – vertical compression.
	Example of treatment – nonspecific (for the sternal fracture).

RIBS (Fig. 8.5)

There are 12 pairs of ribs.

1–7 are true ribs as they are directly attached to the sternum by the costal cartilage.

8–12 are false ribs; 8–10 are indirectly attached to the sternum by their costal cartilages; 11 and 12 are floating ribs as they are not attached to the sternum.

3rd–9th ribs are considered to be 'typical'.

The ribs increase in size from 1–7 and then decrease in size.

In vivo the ribs are inclined downwards and forwards. Therefore the posterior ends are at a higher level than the anterior ends.

Type

Flat bone.

Position

Form the thoracic cage.

Articulations

The anterior end is connected to the sternum by the costal cartilage to form the sternocostal joint.

The head with the demi-facets of the vertebral bodies to form the costovertebral joint.

The articular part of the tubercle with the transverse process of the vertebra to form the costotransverse joint.

Main parts

Anterior end – concavity for the costal cartilage.

Head – forms the posterior end with the neck and tubercle.

Crest – divides the head transversely. On either side are a lower and upper facet for articulation with the vertebral body of the same segment and the one of the segment above.

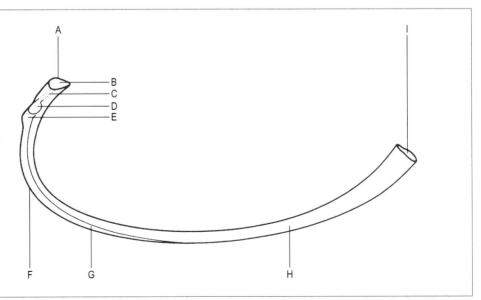

Fig. 8.5 A 'typical' left rib (inferior aspect).
A – Crest
B – Facet of the head
C – Neck
D – Articular part of tubercle
E – Non-articular part of tubercle
F – Angle
G – Costal groove
H – Shaft
I – Anterior end.

Neck – narrow portion below the head; lies in front of the transverse process of the corresponding vertebra.

Tubercle – has a medial articular facet for articulation with the vertebra at the transverse process, and a lateral non-articular facet.

Angle – near the posterior end of the rib.

Shaft – long and flat.

Costal groove – on the inferior border of the internal surface of the shaft; gives attachment to the intercostal muscle and contains intercostal vessels and nerves.

Ossification

Primary centre

Shaft – 8th week intrauterine life.

Secondary centres

3 centres:
head appears at puberty;
articular part of the tubercle appears at puberty;
non-articular part of the tubercle appears at puberty.
Fuse with shaft age 20.

ATYPICAL RIBS

1st rib (Fig. 8.6)

Short, flat and broad.

Head – single articular facet (articulates only with the body of the 1st thoracic vertebra).

Tubercle – wide and prominent.

Costal groove – absent.

Inner border – concave.

Outer border – convex.

Upper surface – has a posterior groove occupied by the subclavian artery and an anterior groove for the subclavian vein with a long ridge between.

Lower surface.

Ossification

Primary centre

Shaft – 8th week intrauterine life.

Secondary centres

2 centres:
head appears at puberty;
tubercle appears at puberty.
Fuse with shaft age 20.

2nd rib (Fig. 8.7)

Approximately twice the length of the 1st rib.

Costal groove – poorly marked.

Rough area – outer surface, for the attachment of the serratus anterior muscle.

Ossification

As for a typical rib.

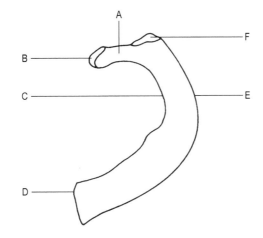

Fig. 8.6 Left 1st rib (superior aspect).
A – Neck
B – Head
C – Inner border
D – Anterior end
E – Outer border
F – Tubercle.

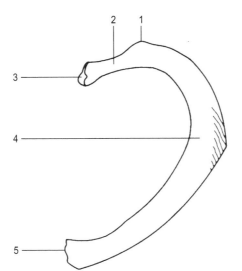

Fig. 8.7 Left 2nd rib (superior aspect).
1 – Tubercle
2 – Neck
3 – Head
4 – Shaft
5 – Anterior end.

10th rib

Has only one facet – for articulation with the 10th thoracic vertebra.

Ossification As for a typical rib.

11th rib

Short.
Has only one facet – for articulation with the 11th thoracic vertebra.
Tubercle – absent.
Neck – absent.

Ossification **Primary centre**
Shaft – 8th week intrauterine life.

Secondary centre
1 centre:
  head appears at puberty.
  Fuses with shaft age 20.

12th rib

Shorter than the 11th rib.
Has only one facet – for articulation with the 12th thoracic vertebra.
Tubercle – absent.
Neck – absent.

Ossification **Primary centre**
Shaft – 8th week intrauterine life.

Secondary centre
1 centre:
  head appears at puberty.
  Fuses with shaft age 20.

Radiographic appearances of the ribs (Figs 8.8, 8.9 and 8.10, Plate 5)

Fig. 8.8 Upper ribs: posterior projection.
(From Bryan 1996.)
A – Clavicle
B – Posterior borders of 4th, 5th and 6th ribs
C – Heart
D – Anterior end of 6th rib
E – Diaphragm
F – 9th rib
G – 8th rib
H – 7th rib
I – 6th rib
J – 5th rib
K – 4th rib
L – Anterior borders of 1st, 2nd and 3rd ribs.

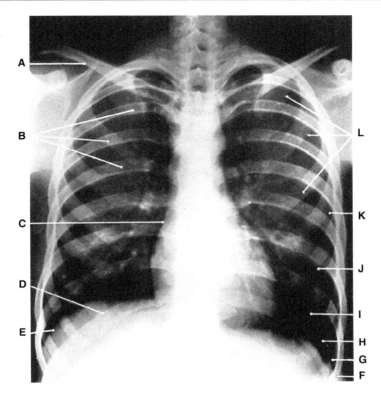

Fig. 8.9 Lower ribs: anteroposterior projection.
(From Bryan 1996.)
1 – Lung tissues
2 – Diaphragm
3 – Diaphragm
4 – Heart.

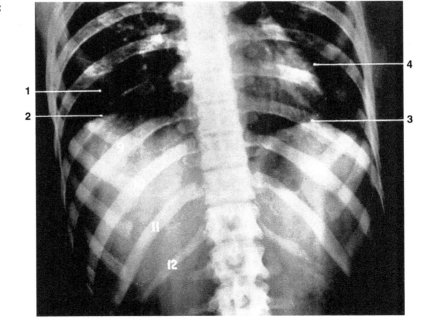

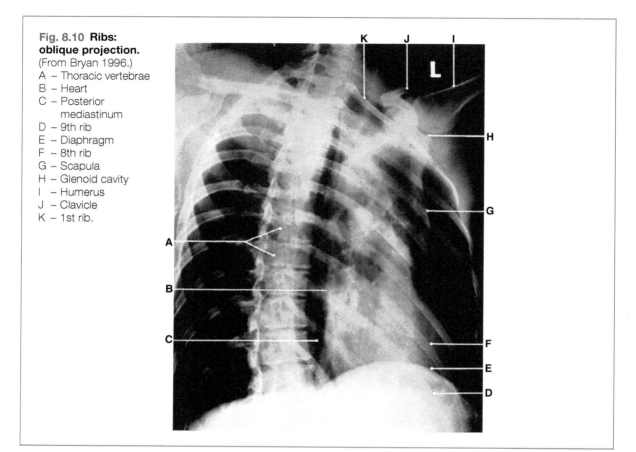

Fig. 8.10 Ribs: oblique projection.
(From Bryan 1996.)
A – Thoracic vertebrae
B – Heart
C – Posterior mediastinum
D – 9th rib
E – Diaphragm
F – 8th rib
G – Scapula
H – Glenoid cavity
I – Humerus
J – Clavicle
K – 1st rib.

COSTAL CARTILAGES (Fig. 8.11)

Formed by hyaline cartilage.
Base is attached to the anterior end of the ribs.
Costal cartilages of the:

1st–7th ribs articulate with the sternum
8th–10th ribs articulate with the costal cartilage of the rib above
11th and 12th ribs end in the muscles of the abdominal wall.

The costal cartilages:

increase in length from the 1st to the 7th
decrease in length from the 8th to the 12th
decrease in width from the 1st to the 12th.

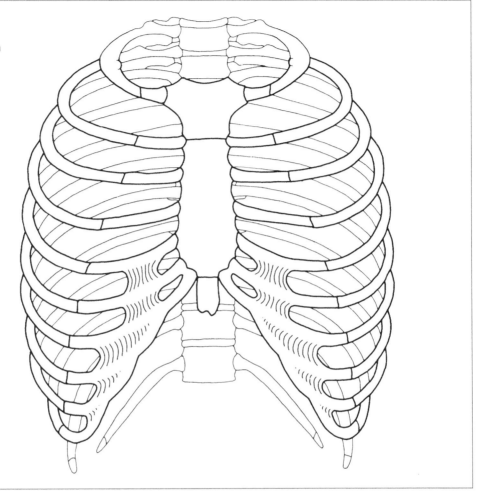

Fig. 8.11 **The bony thorax – demonstrating the position of the costal cartilages.**

Fractures

Usually near the angle

Cause – direct blow.

Example of treatment – non-specific; assist with patient comfort.

N.B. Associated chest injuries may result, for example:

Haemothorax – blood in the pleural cavity.

Pneumothorax – air in the pleural cavity causing lung collapse.

Haemo-pneumothorax – combination of the previous two.

Emphysema – air in the subcutaneous tissue and in planes between the muscles.

Vertebral column | 9

CHAPTER CONTENTS

The vertebral column usually consists of:
  7 cervical vertebrae (movable)
  12 thoracic vertebrae (movable)
  5 lumbar vertebrae (movable)
  5 sacral segments (fused)
  4 coccygeal segments (fused to a variable extent).

A 'TYPICAL' VERTEBRA

INSIGHT

By learning the parts of a typical vertebra, the majority of the parts of the cervical, thoracic and lumbar vertebrae can be identified.

Type   Irregular bone.

Position   Forms part of the central axis of the body.

Articulations   *Superior articular facets* with the inferior articular facets of the vertebra above to form the joints of the vertebral arches.

Inferior articular facets with the superior articular facets of the vertebra below to form the joints of the vertebral arches.

Between the vertebral bodies to form the intervertebral joints.

Main parts

Body – cancellous bone covered with compact bone; anterior surface is convex.

Pedicles – project back from the postero-lateral aspects of the body.

Laminae – project back from the ends of the pedicles; fuse in the midline.

Vertebral arch – formed by 2 pedicles and 2 laminae.

Vertebral foramen – formed by the posterior aspect of the body and the vertebral arch. The vertebral foramina and intervertebral joints and ligaments form the vertebral canal, which transmits and protects the spinal cord, spinal nerve roots and meninges.

Transverse processes – project laterally from the junction of the pedicles and laminae.

Spinous process – projects backwards from the junction of the laminae.

Superior articular processes – projections on the superior aspect of the vertebral arch at the junction of the pedicles and the laminae which carry the superior articular facets.

Inferior articular processes – projections on the inferior aspect of the vertebral arch which carry the inferior articular facets.

Vertebral notches, superior and inferior – formed between the body and the articular processes above and below the pedicles.

Intervertebral foramina – formed by the vertebral notches, between the pedicles of adjacent vertebrae. Transmit the spinal nerves. Lie at an angle of 45° to the median sagittal plane and 0–15° to the horizontal.

Ossification

Primary centres

3 centres.

Body – between the 9th–10th week of intrauterine life and age 4 months.

Vertebral arch (2 centres) – between the 9th week of intrauterine life and age 3 months.

Vertebral arch fuses age 1–6.
Arch fuses with the body at puberty.

Secondary centres

5 centres appear after puberty:

Spinous process – end 1 centre.

Transverse process – 1 centre for each process.

Body – 1 centre upper surface, 1 centre lower surface.

Fuse together age 25.

CERVICAL VERTEBRAE

3rd to 6th (typical) (Figs 9.1 and 9.2)

Features

Size – smaller than the thoracic and lumbar vertebrae.

Body – small, oval in shape.

Lamina – long and thin.

Vertebral foramen – large and triangular (cervical enlargement).

Pedicles – short, round, project laterally and backwards 45°.

Intervertebral foramen – directed forwards and laterally.

Transverse processes – carry the foramen transversarium for the vertebral arteries; these divide the processes into anterior and posterior roots, which end in small tubercles.

Superior articular facet – faces upwards and backwards.

Inferior articular facet – faces downwards and forwards.

Spinous process – short and bifid (divided).

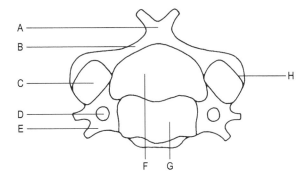

Fig. 9.1 **A typical cervical vertebra (superior aspect).**
A – Spinous process
B – Lamina
C – Superior articular facet
D – Foramen transversarium
E – Transverse process
F – Vertebral foramen
G – Body
H – Superior articular process.

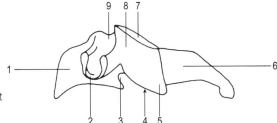

Fig. 9.2 **A typical cervical vertebra (lateral aspect).**
1 – Body
2 – Transverse process
3 – Inferior vertebral notch
4 – Inferior articular facet
5 – Inferior articular process
6 – Spinous process
7 – Superior articular facet
8 – Superior articular process
9 – Superior vertebral notch.

Radiographic appearances of the cervical vertebrae (Figs 9.3, 9.4, 9.5, 9.6 and Plate 6)

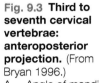

Fig. 9.3 Third to seventh cervical vertebrae: anteroposterior projection. (From Bryan 1996.)

A – Angle of mandible
B – Larynx
C – Body of 5th cervical vertebra
D – Trachea
E – Spinous process of 7th cervical vertebra
F – Body of 1st thoracic vertebra
G – 1st rib
H – Transverse process of 7th cervical vertebra
I – Spinous process
J – Level of vocal folds
K – Transverse process
L – Articular process.

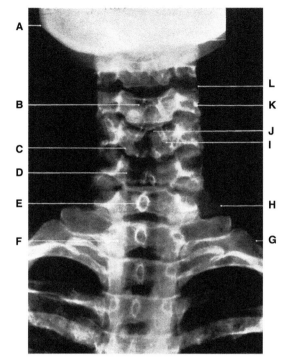

Fig. 9.4 Cervical vertebrae: lateral projection. (From Bryan 1996.)

1 – Anterior tubercle of atlas
2 – Odontoid process
3 – Mandible
4 – Body of 4th cervical vertebra
5 – Transverse process
6 – Body of 1st thoracic vertebra
7 – 1st rib
8 – Pedicle
9 – Spinous process of 7th cervical vertebra (vertebra prominens)
10 – Inferior articular process
11 – Superior articular process
12 – Lamina
13 – Spinous process of axis
14 – Posterior tubercle of atlas
15 – Occipital bone
16 – Atlanto-occipital joint.

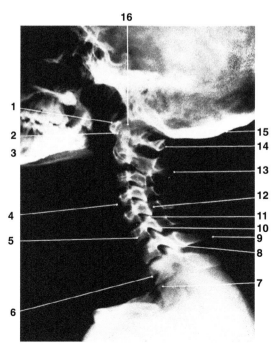

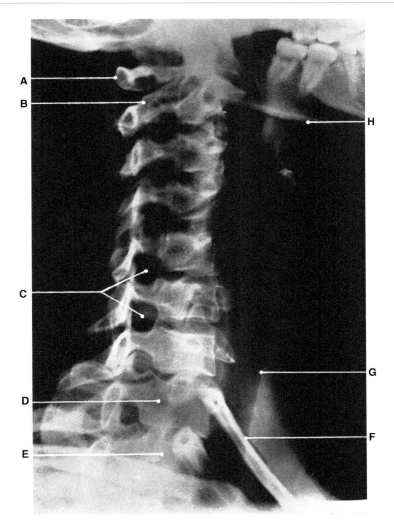

Fig. 9.5 **Cervical vertebrae: oblique anteroposterior projection.** (From Bryan 1996.)

A – Atlas
B – Spinous process of axis
C – Right intervertebral foramina
D – 1st thoracic vertebra
E – 2nd thoracic vertebra
F – 1st rib
G – Trachea
H – Mandible.

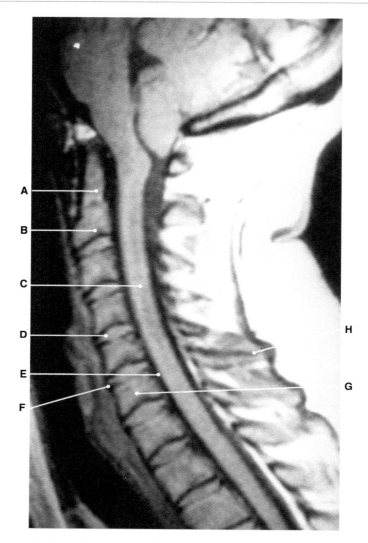

Fig. 9.6 Atlas and axis (C1 and C2): MR scan to cervical vertebrae. (From Bryan 1996.)
A – Odontoid process
B – Body of axis (C2)
C – Spinal cord
D – Intervertebral disc
E – Posterior longitudinal ligament
F – Anterior longitudinal ligament
G – Vertebral body
H – Spinous process of 6th cervical vertebra

1st cervical vertebra (atlas) (Fig. 9.7)

Articulations

Superior articular facets with the occipital condyles to form the atlanto-occipital joints.

Inferior articular facets with the superior articular facets of the 2nd cervical vertebra to form the lateral atlanto-axial joints.

The facet on the anterior arch with the odontoid process of the 2nd cervical vertebra to form the median atlanto-axial joint.

Features

'Ring-shaped' with no body.

Anterior arch – in the midline there is a projection called the anterior tubercle. On the posterior aspect is a facet for the odontoid process of the 2nd cervical vertebra.

Posterior arch – in the midline there is a projection called the posterior tubercle, which represents a rudimentary spinous process. There is a wide groove behind the lateral masses for the vertebral arteries.

Vertebral foramen – oval.

Lateral masses – lie on either side of the vertebral foramen and carry the superior and inferior articular facets. On the medial aspect is a tubercle for the transverse ligament of the atlas.

Superior articular facets – large and oval.

Inferior articular facets – round and flat.

Transverse process – long, assists with rotation of the head.

Foramen transversarium – pierces the transverse process.

Ossification

Primary centres

3 centres:

lateral masses (1 per mass) appear 7th week of intrauterine life;

the masses fuse age 3–4;

anterior arch appears age 1.

Fuse together age 6–8.

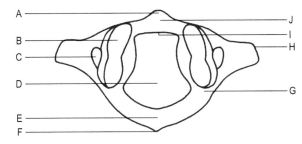

Fig. 9.7 1st cervical vertebra (superior aspect).
A – Anterior tubercle
B – Superior articular facet
C – Foramen transversarium
D – Vertebral foramen
E – Posterior arch
F – Posterior tubercle
G – Groove for the vertebral artery
H – Transverse process
I – Facet for the odontoid process
J – Anterior arch.

2nd cervical vertebra (axis) (Figs 9.8 and 9.9)

Articulations   *Superior articular facets* with the inferior articular facets of the 1st cervical vertebra to form the lateral atlanto-axial joints.
Inferior articular facets with the superior articular facets of the 3rd cervical vertebra to form the joints of the vertebral arches.
The odontoid process with the anterior arch of the 1st cervical vertebra to form the median atlanto-axial joint.
The body with the body of the 3rd cervical vertebra to form the intervertebral joint.

Features   *Odontoid process (dens)* – projection on the upper aspect of the body. Has a facet for articulation with the anterior arch of the 1st cervical vertebra. Represents the body of the atlas.

INSIGHT

Whiplash injuries can cause a fracture of the base of the odontoid process as this is the weakest part of the spine, movement of the head following injury can result in damage to the spinal cord.

Ossification   *Primary centres*
5 centres:
   odontoid process – 2 centres appear 6th month intrauterine life.
   odontoid centres fuse together before birth;
   vertebral arch – 2 centres appear 7th–8th month intrauterine life;
   body – age 4–5 months.

Secondary centres
2 centres:
   odontoid process appears age 2, fuses age 12;
   thin plate under the body appears at puberty.

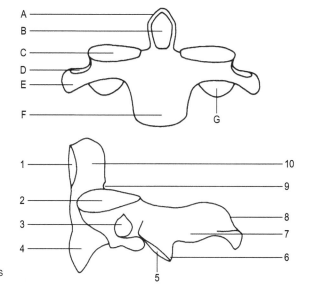

Fig. 9.8 2nd cervical vertebra (axis) (anterior aspect).
A – Odontoid process (dens)
B – Facet for the anterior arch of the atlas
C – Superior articular facet
D – Foramen transversarium
E – Transverse process
F – Body
G – Inferior articular facet.

Fig. 9.9 2nd cervical vertebra (axis) (lateral aspect).
1 – Facet for the anterior arch of the atlas
2 – Superior articular facet
3 – Foramen transversarium
4 – Body
5 – Inferior articular facet
6 – Inferior articular process
7 – Lamina
8 – Spinous process
9 – Groove for the transverse ligament of the atlas
10 – Odontoid process (dens).

Radiographic appearances of the upper cervical vertebrae (Figs 9.10, 9.11 and 9.12)

Fig. 9.10 Upper cervical vertebrae: anteroposterior projection (with mouth open).
(From Bryan 1996.)
A – Lateral mass of atlas
B – Atlanto-axial joint
C – Spinous process of axis
D – 3rd cervical vertebra
E – Mandible
F – Odontoid process.

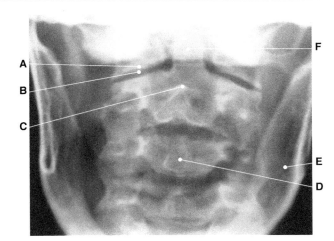

Fig. 9.11 Upper cervical spine: CT scan. (From Bryan 1996.)
1 – Atlanto-occipital joint
2 – Atlanto-axial joint
3 – Body of axis (C2)
4 – Odontoid process
5 – Atlas (C1)
6 – External auditory meatus.

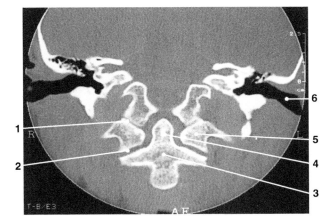

Fig. 9.12 Calcification below the anterior arch of C1 (arrowed). CT scan. (From Resnick Kransdorf, 2005.)

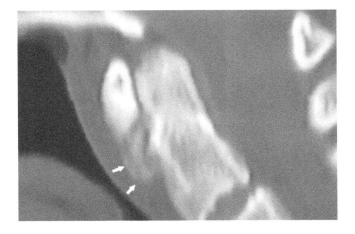

7th cervical vertebra (vertebra prominens)

Spinous process – long, not bifid; useful bony landmark.

Foramina transversarium – rudimentary or absent; vertebral vessels do not pass through them.

Transverse processes – large, may develop a cervical rib.

Ossification

As per a typical vertebra.

2 additional centres for the costal part of the transverse process – appears 6 months intrauterine.

Centres usually fuse age 5–6.

N.B. They may not fuse and can go on to form cervical ribs.

THORACIC VERTEBRAE

2nd to 8th (typical) (Figs 9.13 and 9.14)

Features

INSIGHT

Remember the thoracic body lies near the heart and is heart shaped.

Size – larger than the cervical and smaller than the lumbar vertebrae.

Body – heart-shaped. On either side are 2 demi-facets; the superior demi-facets are larger and lie at the root of the pedicle, and the inferior demi-facets lie on the lower border. All 4 costal facets articulate with the heads of the ribs, the superior with the corresponding rib and the inferior with the one below.

Laminae – short and deep, overlapping those of the vertebra below.

Vertebral foramen – small and circular.

Pedicles – very short, directed backwards. There is virtually no superior vertebral notch.

Transverse processes – thick and strong. Anteriorly there is an oval facet for articulation with the tubercle of the rib.

Superior articular facets – vertical, face backwards.

Inferior articular facets – vertical, face forwards.

Spinous process – long, slender and directed downwards and backwards.

Fig. 9.13 A typical thoracic vertebra (superior aspect).
A – Spinous process
B – Transverse process
C – Superior articular facet
D – Vertebral foramen
E – Body
F – Pedicle
G – Costal facet for the tubercle of the rib
H – Lamina.

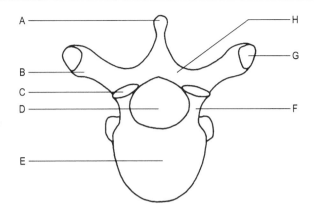

Fig. 9.14 A typical thoracic vertebra (lateral aspect).
1 – Body
2 – Demi-facet for the head of the rib
3 – Inferior vertebral notch
4 – Inferior articular process
5 – Spinous process
6 – Transverse process
7 – Costal facet for the tubercle of the rib
8 – Superior articular facet
9 – Superior articular process
10 – Demi-facet for the head of the rib.

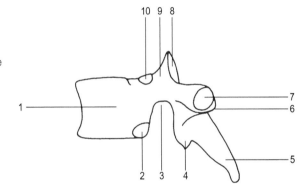

Radiographic appearances of the thoracic vertebrae (Figs 9.15, 9.16 and 9.17)

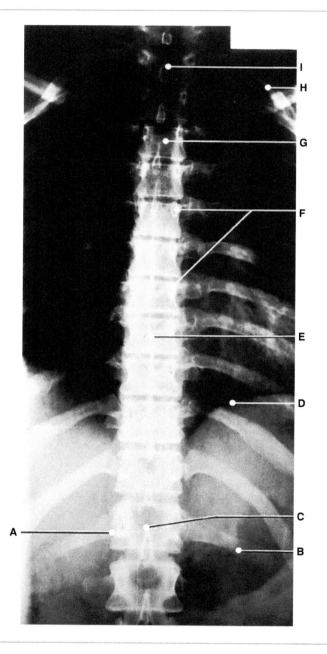

Fig. 9.15 **Thoracic vertebrae: anteroposterior projection.** (From Bryan 1996.)

A – Costovertebral joint
B – 12th rib
C – Body of 12th thoracic vertebra
D – Left dome of diaphragm
E – Spinous process
F – Pedicles
G – Trachea
H – 1st rib
I – Body of 1st thoracic vertebra.

Fig. 9.16 Thoracic vertebrae: lateral projection. (From Bryan 1996.)
1 – Body of 3rd thoracic vertebra
2 – Scapulae
3 – Sternum
4 – Heart
5 – Diaphragm
6 – Body of 12th thoracic vertebra
7 – 12th pair of ribs
8 – Superior articular process
9 – Inferior articular process
10 – Spinous process
11 – Pedicle
12 – Intervertebral foramen.

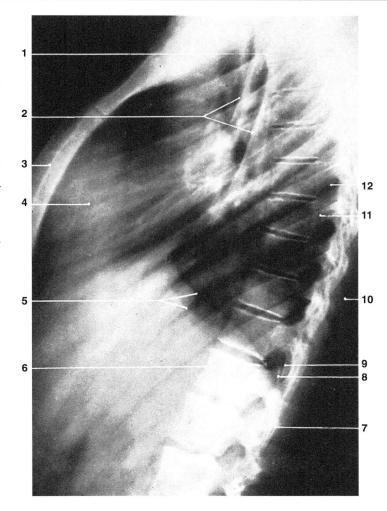

Fig. 9.17 Thoracic vertebra: CT scan. (From Bryan 1996.)
A – Lung
B – Transverse process
C – Spinous process
D – Rib
E – Costovertebral joint
F – Neural canal
G – Vertebral body.

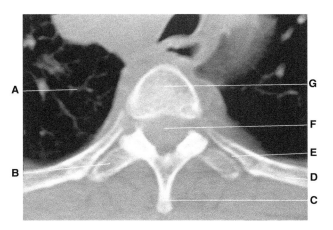

1st thoracic vertebra

Special features   *Body* – full superior costal facets are circular and articulate with the 1st ribs; inferior costal demi-facets are semicircular and articulate with the 2nd ribs.

Spinous process – thick, long and horizontal.

9th thoracic vertebra

Special features   *Body* – inferior costal demi-facets are sometimes absent.

10th thoracic vertebra

Special features   *Body* – sometimes full superior costal facets, oval in shape for articulation with the 10th ribs.

Inferior costal facets – absent.

Transverse processes – facet for articulation with the 10th rib may be absent.

11th thoracic vertebra

Special features   *Body* – full superior costal facets, oval in shape for articulation with the 11th ribs.

Inferior costal facets – absent.

Transverse processes – small, no costal facets.

12th thoracic vertebra

Special features   *Body* – full superior costal facets, lower down, oval in shape for articulation with the 12th ribs.

Inferior costal facets – absent.

Transverse processes – small, no costal facets.

LUMBAR VERTEBRAE

1st to 4th (typical) (Figs 9.18 and 9.19)

Features

INSIGHT

Remember the lumbar body lies near the kidneys and is kidney-shaped.

Fig. 9.18 A typical lumbar vertebra (superior aspect).
A – Spinous process
B – Superior articular process
C – Transverse process
D – Pedicle
E – Body
F – Vertebral foramen
G – Superior articular facet
H – Lamina.

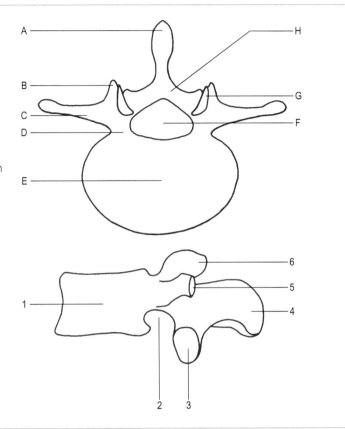

Fig. 9.19 A typical lumbar vertebra (lateral aspect).
1 – Body
2 – Inferior vertebral notch
3 – Inferior articular facet
4 – Spinous process
5 – Transverse process
6 – Superior articular process.

Size – larger than the cervical and thoracic vertebrae.

Body – large and kidney-shaped.

Laminae – short and thick, inclined downwards.

Vertebral foramen – triangular, smaller than the cervical and larger than the thoracic.

Pedicles – short and thick, set on the upper half of the body.

Transverse processes – long and thin.

Superior articular processes – have a rough elevation on the posterior border called the mamillary process.

Superior articular facets – vertical, facing medially and posteriorly.

Inferior articular facets – vertical, facing laterally and anteriorly.

Pars interarticularis – between the superior and inferior articular processes. Deficient in spondylolisthesis. Demonstrated radiographically in the oblique projection.

Spinous process – quadrilateral in shape, thickened on the posterior and inferior margins.

Accessory transverse process – found at the inferior aspect of the root of the transverse process.

Ossification

Primary centres

3 centres:

body – appears between 9th to 10th week of intrauterine life and age 4 months;

vertebral arch (2 centres) – appears between the 9th week of intrauterine life and age 3 months.

Vertebral arch fuses age 1–6.

Arch fuses with the body at puberty.

Secondary centres

7 centres appear after puberty:

spinous process – end 1 centre;

transverse process – 1 centre for each process;

body – 1 centre upper surface, 1 centre lower surface;

mamillary process – 1 centre per process, appears at puberty.

Fuse together age 25.

Radiographic appearances of the lumbar vertebrae (Figs 9.20, 9.21, 9.22 and 9.23)

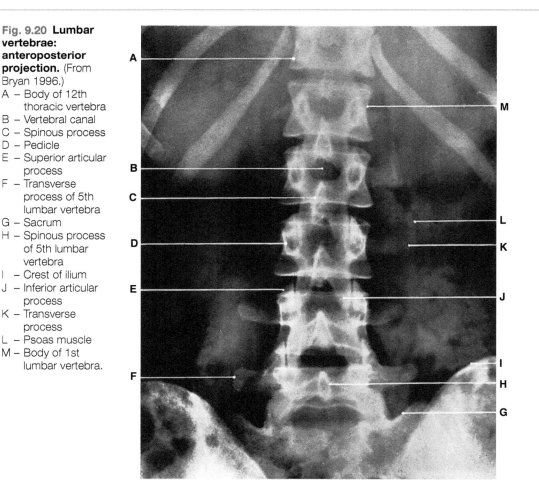

Fig. 9.20 **Lumbar vertebrae: anteroposterior projection.** (From Bryan 1996.)

A – Body of 12th thoracic vertebra

B – Vertebral canal

C – Spinous process

D – Pedicle

E – Superior articular process

F – Transverse process of 5th lumbar vertebra

G – Sacrum

H – Spinous process of 5th lumbar vertebra

I – Crest of ilium

J – Inferior articular process

K – Transverse process

L – Psoas muscle

M – Body of 1st lumbar vertebra.

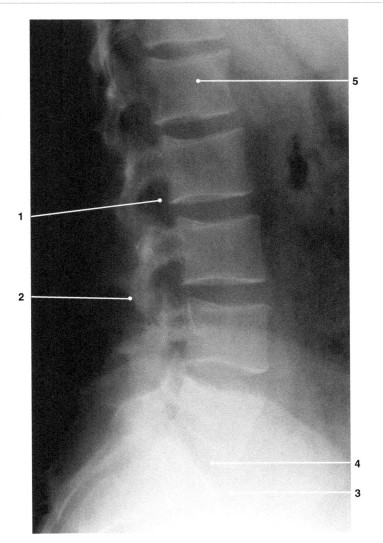

Fig. 9.21 Lumbar vertebrae: lateral projection. (From Bryan 1996.)
1 – Intervertebral foramen
2 – Spinous process
3 – Sacral promontory
4 – Lumbosacral joint
5 – Body of 1st lumbar vertebra.

5th lumbar vertebra

Special features   *Body* – largest of all vertebrae, deeper anteriorly than posteriorly.

Transverse processes – large, connected to the whole of the pedicle and part of the body.

Fig. 9.22 Lumbar vertebrae: left posterior oblique projection.
(From Bryan 1996.)
A – Right transverse process
B – Superior right articular process
C – Inferior right articular process
D – Left joint space
E – Lamina
F – Spinous process
G – Sacroiliac joint
H – Body of 5th lumbar vertebra
I – Pars interarticularis
J – Left inferior articular process
K – Left transverse process
L – Left superior articular process
M – Pedicle
N – Left 12th rib.

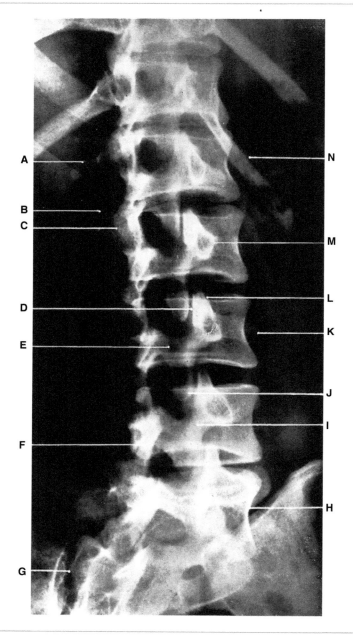

INSIGHT

To check the patient is positioned correctly look for the 'Scotty dog' on the spinal body.

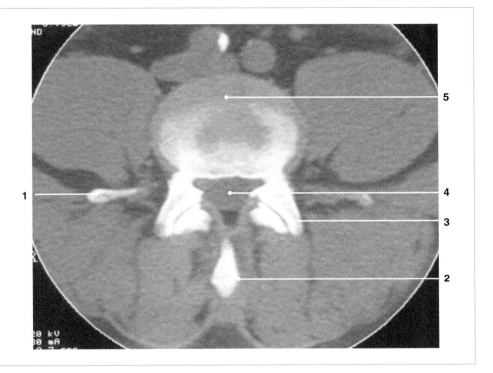

Fig. 9.23 Lumbar spine: CT scan.
(From Bryan 1996.)
1 – Transverse process
2 – Spinous process
3 – Facet joint
4 – Spinal canal
5 – Vertebral body.

SACRUM (Figs 9.24 and 9.25)

The sacrum is composed of 5 sacral segments, which are fused together to form a single bone.

Type   Irregular bone.

Position   Forms the posterior part of the pelvic girdle, between the hip bones.

Articulations   *The base* articulates with the body of the 5th lumbar vertebra to form the lumbosacral joint.
The apex articulates with the base of the coccyx to form the sacrococcygeal joint.
The auricular facet articulates with the auricular surface of the hip bone to form the sacroiliac joint.

Main parts   **Base**
This is formed by the 1st sacral segment and has the following features:
Body – large and wide; anterior edge is called the sacral promontory.
Laminae – inclined downwards, medially and posteriorly.

Pedicles – short; face posteriorly and laterally.

Transverse processes – project from the body, pedicles and superior articular processes; are fused with the costal element to form the lateral surface, the ala.

Superior articular facets – vertical; face medially and posteriorly.

Spinous tubercle – small spinous process.

Pelvic surface

This faces inferiorly and anteriorly, is concave and relatively smooth, and has the following features:

Pelvic sacral foramina – 4 pairs which carry the first 4 sacral spinal nerves from the sacral canal.

Transverse ridges – 4 ridges between the pelvic sacral foramina, denoting the fusion of the vertebral bodies.

Costal elements – formed by the area between the pelvic sacral foramina, and lateral to them, where the costal elements are fused with the transverse processes.

Dorsal surface

This faces superiorly and posteriorly, is convex and has the following features:

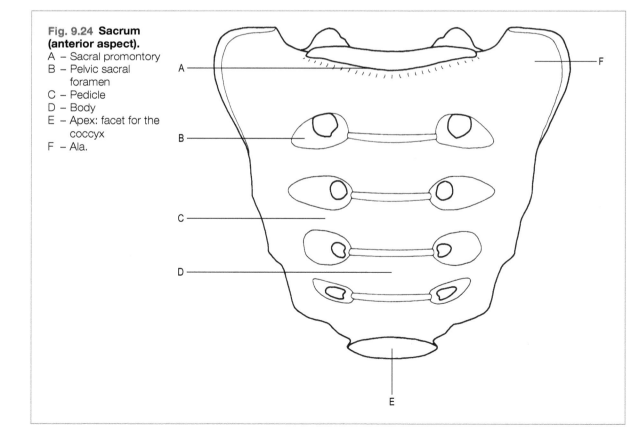

Fig. 9.24 Sacrum (anterior aspect).
A – Sacral promontory
B – Pelvic sacral foramen
C – Pedicle
D – Body
E – Apex: facet for the coccyx
F – Ala.

Medial sacral crest – raised promontory of bone in the midline representing the fused spinous processes.

Spinous tubercles – 4 (sometimes 3) tubercles on the crest.

Sacral hiatus – the laminae of the 5th sacral segment fail to meet in the midline, forming a gap in the posterior wall of sacral canal.

Dorsal sacral foramina – four pairs of foramina which carry the first four dorsal sacral nerves from the sacral canal.

Intermediate sacral crests – each crest is formed by 4 tubercles and lies medial to the dorsal sacral foramina, representing the fused articular processes.

Sacral cornua – formed by the inferior articular processes of the 5th sacral segment, and lie either side of the sacral hiatus.

Lateral sacral crests – formed by the fused transverse processes, lateral to the dorsal sacral foramina.

Transverse tubercles – a row of tubercles on the lateral sacral crests.

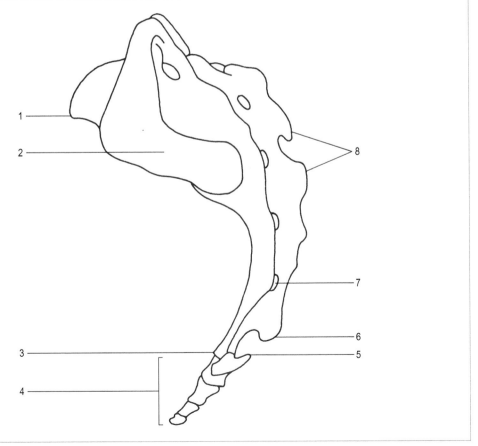

Fig. 9.25 Sacrum (lateral aspect).
1 – Sacral promontory
2 – Auricular facet
3 – Sacrococcygeal joint
4 – Coccyx
5 – Coccygeal cornu
6 – Sacral cornu
7 – Dorsal sacral foramen
8 – Spinous tubercles.

Lateral surface

Triangular, with the following features:

Auricular facet – 'ear-shaped' surface for articulation with the ilium.

Lateral border – thin, lies below the auricular surface.

Inferior lateral angle – towards the lower end of the lateral border at the level of the 5th segment.

Apex

The inferior aspect of the 5th sacral segment. It has the following feature:

Oval facet – for articulation with the coccyx.

Sacral canal

Triangular, formed by the vertebral foramina.

The upper opening lies obliquely and the canal terminates at the sacral hiatus.

Ossification (for each of the vertebral segments.)

Primary centres

Costal elements – appear 6th–8th month intrauterine life.

Vertebral arch (2 centres) – appear age 10–12 weeks.
    Costal elements fuse age 2–5.
    Vertebral arches fuse at puberty.
    Arch fuses with the body at puberty.

Secondary centres

Centres appear after puberty:
    spinous tubercle – end 1 centre;
    transverse process – 1 centre for each process;
    body – 1 centre upper surface, 1 centre lower surface;
    costal epiphyseal centres – 6 centres.
    Fuse together age 20.

Radiographic appearances of the sacrum (Figs 9.26, 9.27, 9.28 and 9.29)

Fig. 9.26 **Sacrum: anteroposterior projection.**
(From Bryan 1996.)
A – Superior articular process of 1st segment
B – Ala of sacrum
C – Spinous tubercle
D – Intervertebral foramina
E – Sacral hiatus
F – Pelvic brim
G – Symphysis pubis
H – Coccyx
I – Sacrococcygeal joint
J – Inferior angle
K – Articular tubercle
L – Transverse tubercle
M – Sacroiliac joint
N – Ilium
O – Body of 1st sacral segment
P – Lumbosacral joint
Q – Spinous process of 5th lumbar vertebra.

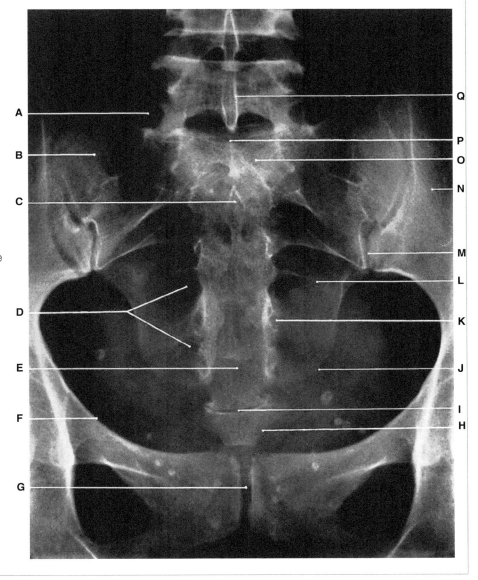

Fig. 9.27 Sacrum and coccyx: lateral projection. (From Bryan 1996.)

1 – Superior articular process
2 – Sacrum
3 – Sacral canal
4 – Spinous tubercles
5 – Gas in rectum
6 – Coccyx
7 – Sacral promontory
8 – Lumbosacral joint
9 – 5th lumbar vertebra.

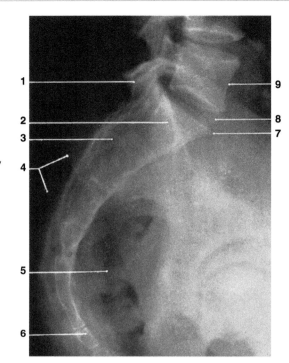

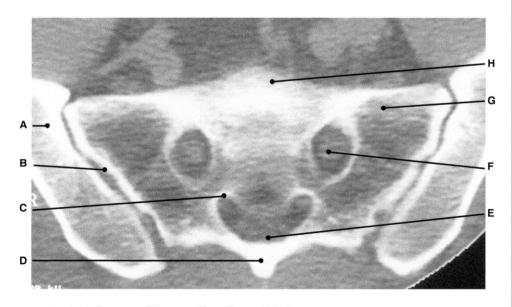

Fig. 9.28 Sacrum: CT scan. (From Bryan 1996.)

A – Ilium
B – Sacroiliac joint
C – Margin of sacral foramen
D – Spinous tubercle
E – Sacral canal
F – Anterior sacral foramen
G – Lateral mass of sacrum
H – Sacral promontory.

Fig. 9.29 Sacral fracture (arrowed). CT scan.
(From Resnick Kransdorf, 2005.)

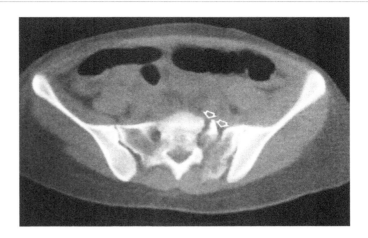

COCCYX (Fig. 9.30)

The coccyx is composed of between 3 and 5 segments, partly or totally fused together to form a triangular bone.

Type

Irregular bone.

Position

Lies on the inferior aspect of the sacrum in the midline and forms the base of the spine.

Articulations

The base articulates with the apex of the sacrum to form the sacrococcygeal joint.

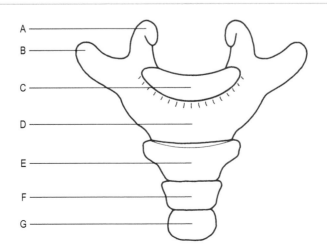

Fig. 9.30 Coccyx (anterior aspect).
A – Coccygeal cornu
B – Rudimentary transverse process
C – Facet for the sacrum
D – 1st coccygeal segment
E – 2nd coccygeal segment
F – 3rd coccygeal segment
G – 4th coccygeal segment.

Main parts

Base – formed by the upper surface of the first coccygeal segment; has an oval facet for articulation with the sacrum.

Coccygeal cornua – project upwards.

Transverse processes – rudimentary; from the body of the 1st coccygeal segment.

2nd to 4th segments – diminish in size and represent rudimentary vertebral bodies.

Ossification

Primary centres

Body – 1 centre per body, 1st present at birth.
 Rest appear up to age 20.
 Fuse together up to age 30.

Radiographic appearances of the coccyx (Fig. 9.31)

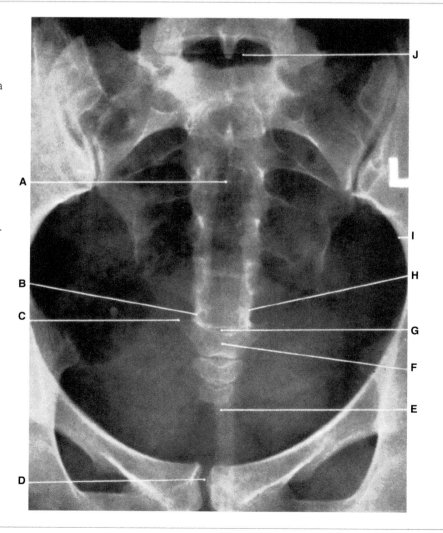

Fig. 9.31 **Coccyx: anteroposterior projection.** (From Bryan 1996.)
A – Sacrum
B – Coccygeal cornua
C – Transverse process
D – Symphysis pubis
E – 4th segment
F – Coccyx 1st segment
G – Sacrococcygeal joint
H – Sacral cornua
I – Pelvic brim
J – Lumbosacral joint.

VERTEBRAL CURVATURES (Fig. 9.32)

The curves of the spinal column can be divided into primary and secondary curves.

Fetus

Presents with two primary curves:

Thoracic curve – concave forwards.

Pelvic curve – concave forwards.

Development of secondary curves

Cervical curve – convex; accentuated when the child begins to hold its head up and when it sits upright at 3–6 months.

Lumbar curve – convex; appears when the child begins to walk at 12–18 months.

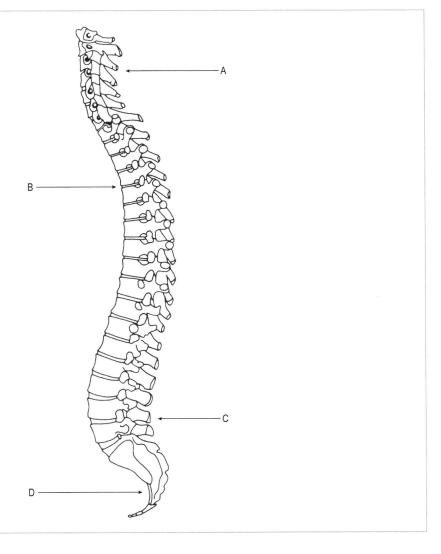

Fig. 9.32 Vertebral column (lateral aspect).
A – Secondary curve, cervical
B – Primary curve, thoracic
C – Secondary curve, lumbar
D – Primary curve, pelvic (sacrococcygeal).

Adult	Presents with four curves:
	Cervical – slightly convex, secondary.
	Thoracic – concave, primary.
	Lumbar – convex, secondary.
	Pelvic – concave, primary.

JOINTS OF THE VERTEBRAL COLUMN

Atlanto-occipital joints

Type	Synovial ellipsoid joints.
Bony articular surfaces	Superior articular facets of the atlas with the condyles of the occipital bone. Both surfaces are covered with articular hyaline cartilage.
Fibrous capsule	Surrounds the condyles of the occipital bone and the superior articular facets of the atlas; is sometimes absent medially.
Synovial membrane	Lines the fibrous capsule and secretes synovial fluid, which lubricates the joint. May communicate with the synovial bursa between the odontoid process and the transverse ligament of the atlas.
Supporting membranes	*Anterior atlanto-occipital membrane* –from the anterior margins of the foramen magnum to the anterior arch of the atlas.
	Posterior atlanto-occipital membrane – from the posterior margins of the foramen magnum to the posterior arch of the atlas.
Movements	*Flexion/extension* – nodding of the head.
	Lateral flexion.

Median atlanto-axial joint

Type	Synovial pivot joint.
Bony articular surfaces	Odontoid process of the axis and the anterior arch of the atlas. Both surfaces are covered with articular hyaline cartilage.
Fibrous capsule	Surrounds the odontoid process of the axis and the facet on the arch of the atlas. It is weak and loose.
Synovial membrane	Lines the fibrous capsule and the bursa and secretes synovial fluid, which lubricates the joint. Posteriorly is a bursa between the anterior surface of the transverse ligament and the posterior surface of the odontoid process.
Strengthening ligaments	*Transverse ligament of the atlas* – maintains the odontoid process in contact with the anterior arch of the atlas.
Movements	*Rotation* – shaking of the head.

Intervertebral joints (Fig. 9.33)

Type	Cartilaginous symphyses.
Bony articular surfaces	The upper and lower surfaces of the respective vertebral bodies. Both surfaces are covered with articular hyaline cartilage recessed within a peripheral non-articular strip.
Strengthening ligaments	*Anterior longitudinal ligament* – extends from the basilar part of the occipital bone to the anterior aspect of the sacrum. It is attached to the intervertebral discs and the margins of the vertebral bodies.
	Posterior longitudinal ligament – extends from the body of the axis to the posterior aspect of the sacrum. It is attached to the intervertebral discs and the margins of the vertebral bodies.
Intracapsular structures	*Intervertebral disc* – consists of an outer portion, the annulus fibrosus, and an inner core, the nucleus pulposus, which is nearer the posterior aspect; therefore the annulus is thinner and weaker behind than in front.
Movements	Individually allow a limited degree of:
	Flexion.
	Extension.
	Lateral flexion.
	Rotation.
	Summated over the length of the spinal column the movement is considerable.

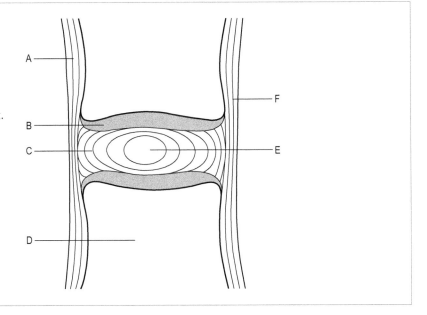

Fig. 9.33 Intervertebral joint (sagittal section).
A – Anterior longitudinal ligament
B – Articular hyaline cartilage
C – Annulus fibrosus
D – Vertebral body
E – Nucleus pulposus
F – Posterior longitudinal ligament.

Radiographic appearances of the ligaments of the vertebral column (Fig. 9.34)

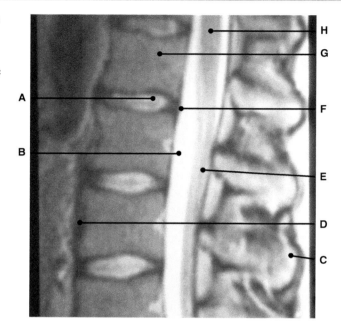

Fig. 9.34 Ligaments of the vertebral column: MR scan.
(From Bryan 1996.)
A – Intervertebral disc
B – Spinal canal
C – Spinous process
D – Anterior longitudinal ligament
E – Cauda equina
F – Posterior longitudinal ligament
G – Vertebral body
H – Conus medullaris

JOINTS OF THE VERTEBRAL ARCHES

Type	Synovial plane joints.
Bony articular surfaces	Superior articular facet with the inferior articular facet of the vertebra above. Both surfaces are covered with articular hyaline cartilage.
Fibrous capsule	Thin, loose and attached to the margins of the articular facets.
Synovial membrane	Lines the fibrous capsule and secretes synovial fluid, which lubricates the joint.
Strengthening ligaments	*Supraspinous ligament* – connects spinous processes.
	Interspinous ligaments – connect adjoining spines.
	Ligamentum nuchae – corresponds to the supraspinous and interspinous ligaments of the cervical region, from the external occipital protuberance and crest to the 7th cervical spinous process.
	Intertransverse ligaments – connect the transverse processes.
	Ligamento flava – connects adjoining laminae.
Movements	*Gliding.*

COSTOVERTEBRAL JOINTS

Type	Synovial plane joints.
Bony articular surfaces	Head of the rib with the facets on the adjoining vertebrae. Both surfaces are covered with articular hyaline cartilage.
Fibrous capsule	Surrounds the head of the rib and the margins of the costal facets of the vertebrae.
Synovial membrane	Lines the fibrous capsule and secretes synovial fluid, which lubricates the joint.
Strengthening ligaments	*Intra-articular ligament* – divides the joint into 2 halves. *Radiate ligament.*

Trauma

INSIGHT

If the spinal cord is damaged due to trauma of the spine there is a danger of paralysis below the area of damage.

Articular processes (Fig. 9.35)

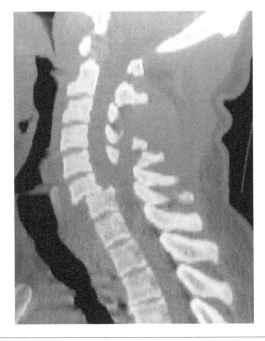

Fig. 9.35 **Fracture dislocation C6–C7, fractures of the C6 laminae.** (From Resnick Kransdorf, 2005.)

Can cause a fracture – dislocation; therefore there is a danger of paraplegia or quadriplegia below the level of the fracture.

Cause – crushing, e.g. mining accidents.

Examples of treatment – Cervical region; traction via skull calipers. Thoracic region: if no injury to spinal cord, plaster jacket; if injury to spinal cord, treatment for paraplegia and rehabilitation. Lumbar region: if no injury or partial damage to spinal cord, internal fixation with metal plate or stainless steel wires; if the cord is severed, treatment for paraplegia and rehabilitation.

Spinous process

The 7th cervical/1st thoracic vertebrae is the most common site.

Cause – direct violence, e.g. a heavy blow.

Example of treatment – rest.

Transverse process

The lumbar spine is the most common site.

Cause – muscular action, e.g. heavy shovelling.

Example of treatment – bed rest.

Vertebral bodies
(Figs 9.36 and 9.37)

Usually a wedge, compression fracture.

Cause – severe flexion, a drop onto the feet or the base of the spine, parachute injury.

Examples of treatment – Cervical region: neck support. Thoracic and lumbar region: bed rest.

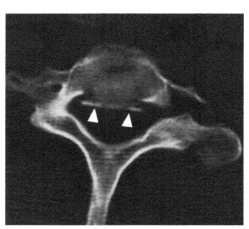

Fig. 9.36 Fracture of the body of C7 (arrowed). CT scan. (From Resnick Kransdorf, 2005.)

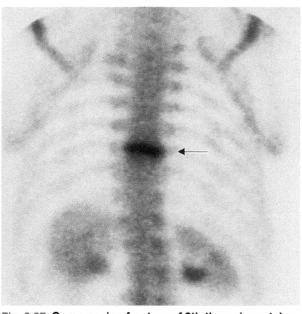

Fig. 9.37 Compression fracture of 9th thoracic vertebra. Radionuclide imaging. (From Resnick Kransdorf, 2005.)

Dislocation

The cervical spine is most common. There is danger of damage to the spinal cord, therefore careful handling is essential.

Cause – whiplash injury: car driver's (or passenger's) head goes forward and then back quickly.

Example of treatment – traction via skull calipers.

Pathology

Cervical rib

An additional rib from the 7th cervical vertebra. Surgical removal is indicated if it causes pressure on the subclavian artery or the brachial nerve plexus; the latter results in loss of sensation along the medial border of the forearm and wasting of the small muscles of the hand.

Schmorl's nodes (Fig. 9.38)

Erosion of the bodies of the vertebrae due to pressure from the nucleus pulposus. It may result in narrowing of the disc space.

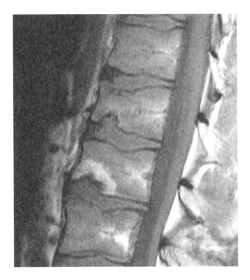

Fig. 9.38 **Schmorl's nodes and multiple degenerative discs. MR scan.** (From Resnick Kransdorf, 2005.)

Lordosis

Excessive secondary curvature, usually in the lumbar region.

Spina bifida

Abnormality of the vertebral arch, which is incomplete posteriorly because of failure of fusion of the laminae.

Spina bifida cystica – protrusion of the meninges or meninges and spinal cord through the defect.

Spondylolisthesis

The moving forward of part of one vertebra on another owing to a defect or failure in the pars articularis. The body, pedicles, transverse and superior articular processes separate from the rest of the vertebral arch and slide forwards.

Facet disease (Plate 7)	Degeneration of the joints of the vertebral arch
Scoliosis (Fig. 9.39)	Abnormal lateral curvature of the spine with, in severe cases, rotation of the vertebrae. Vertebral bodies become wedge-shaped.

Fig. 9.39 Scoliosis. Note disc space narrowing, osteophyte formation, vertebral sclerosis and lateral vertebral subluxation. (From Resnick Kransdorf, 2005.)

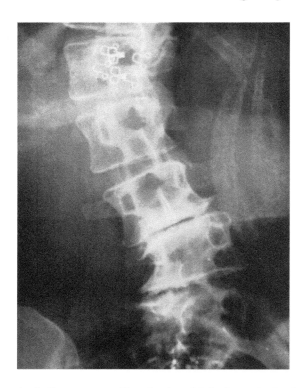

Ankylosing spondylitis (Fig. 9.40)	An inflammatory disorder in which the articular hyaline cartilage is destroyed, the bones fuse and the spinal ligaments ossify. It usually commences in the sacroiliac joints and progresses upwards. Radiographically it is described as a 'bamboo spine'.
Disc degeneration (Fig. 9.41)	Can result in a prolapsed intervertebral disc, which is a protrusion of the nucleus pulposus through a tear in the annulus fibrosus, always posterior or postero-lateral. It may cause pressure on the spinal nerves in the vertebral canal or in the intervertebral foramen: *Lumbago* – pain in the lumbar region. *Sciatica* – pain in the distribution of the sciatic nerve. It is demonstrated during radiculography, discography or CT scanning. *Example of treatment* – manipulation, traction and immobilisation.
Kyphosis	Abnormal flexion of the spine. *Senile kyphosis* – results from disc degeneration causing ossification between the vertebral bodies. *Adolescent kyphosis (Scheuermann's disease)* – disc herniation causes narrowing of the disc spaces, causing the vertebral bodies to tilt forward and impairing normal growth. Result in wedge-shaped vertebral bodies (Figs 9.42 and 9.43).

Fig. 9.40 Ankylosing spondylitis, lumbar spine. (Courtesy of Ernest Higginbottom.)

Fig. 9.41 Disc degeneration, cervical spine. Note the narrowing of the joint spaces and the lipping of the adjacent vertebral bodies. (Courtesy of Ernest Higginbottom.)

Fig. 9.42 Adolescent kyphosis, thoracolumbar spine. (Courtesy of Ernest Higginbottom.)

Fig. 9.43 Scheuermann's disease thoracic spine. (From Resnick Kransdorf, 2005.)

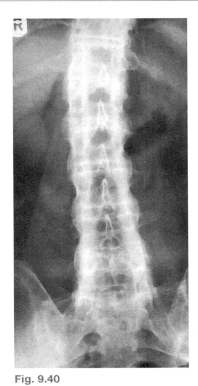

Fig. 9.40

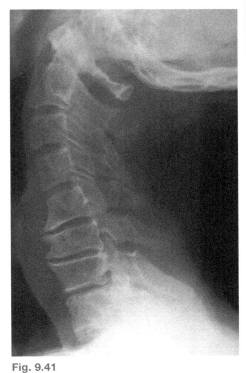

Fig. 9.41

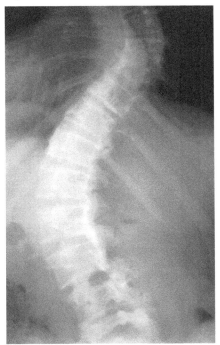

Fig. 9.42

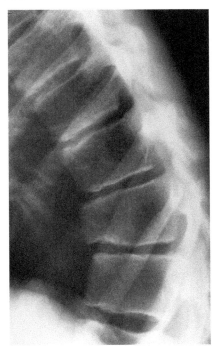

Fig. 9.43

Osteoarthritis
(Fig. 9.44)

Worn articular hyaline cartilage and the formation of osteophytes (bony spurs round the joint margins).

Spondylosis
(Fig. 9.45, Plate 8)

The formation of bony spurs at the disc margins of the vertebral bodies; causes degenerative changes in the intervertebral discs.

Spondylitis

Inflammation of more than one vertebra.

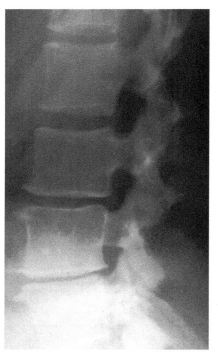

Fig. 9.44 **Osteoarthritis, lumbar spine.**
(Courtesy of Ernest Higginbottom.)

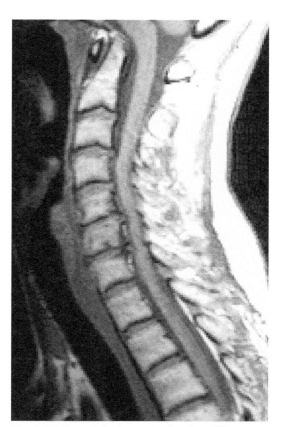

Fig. 9.45 **Spondylosis cervical spine. MR scan.**
(From Resnick Kransdorf, 2005.)

The skull

CHAPTER CONTENTS

SKULL

The skull can be divided into 2 sections: the cranium and the face (Figs 10.1, 10.2 and 10.3).

The cranium is composed of the following bones:

- Occipital bone
- Sphenoid bone
- Temporal bones (2)
- Parietal bones (2)
- Frontal bone
- Ethmoid bone.

The facial bones include:

- Maxillae (2)
- Mandible
- Inferior nasal conchae (2)
- Lacrimal bones (2)
- Nasal bones (2)
- Vomer
- Palatine bones (2)
- Zygomatic bones (2).

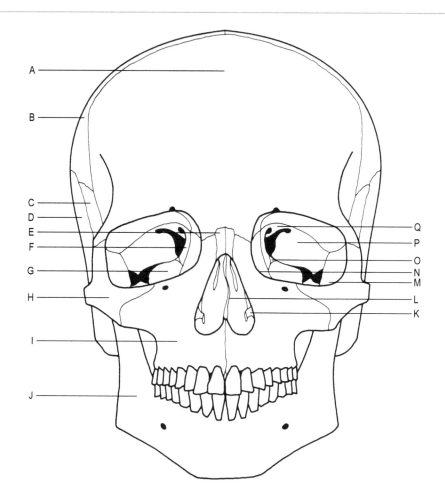

Fig. 10.1 Position of the bones of the skull (anterior aspect).
A – Frontal bone
B – Parietal bone
C – Greater wing of sphenoid bone
D – Temporal bone
E – Nasal bone
F – Ethmoid bone
G – Maxilla
H – Zygomatic bone
I – Maxilla
J – Mandible
K – Inferior nasal concha
L – Vomer
M – Zygomatic bone
N – Lacrimal bone
O – Palatine bone
P – Greater wing of sphenoid bone
Q – Lesser wing of sphenoid bone.

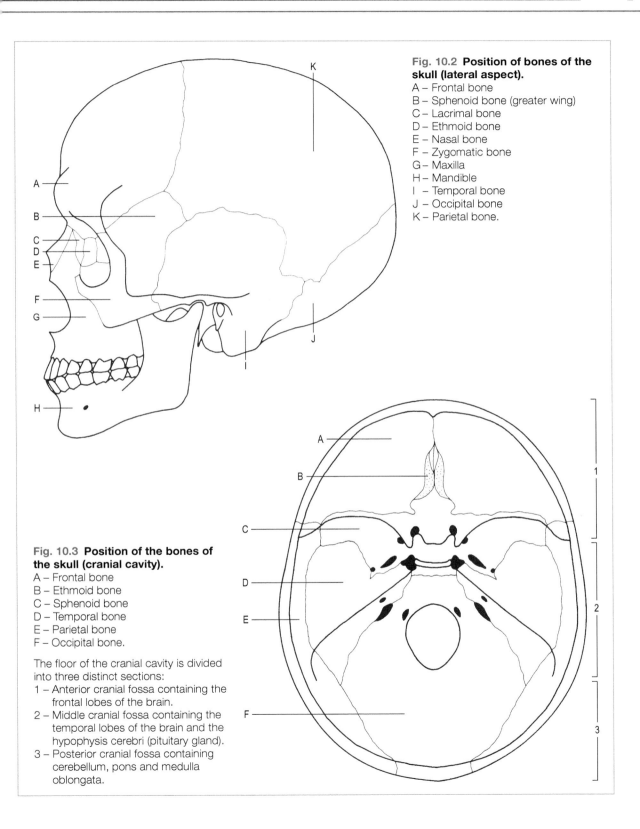

Fig. 10.2 Position of bones of the skull (lateral aspect).
A – Frontal bone
B – Sphenoid bone (greater wing)
C – Lacrimal bone
D – Ethmoid bone
E – Nasal bone
F – Zygomatic bone
G – Maxilla
H – Mandible
I – Temporal bone
J – Occipital bone
K – Parietal bone.

Fig. 10.3 Position of the bones of the skull (cranial cavity).
A – Frontal bone
B – Ethmoid bone
C – Sphenoid bone
D – Temporal bone
E – Parietal bone
F – Occipital bone.

The floor of the cranial cavity is divided into three distinct sections:
1 – Anterior cranial fossa containing the frontal lobes of the brain.
2 – Middle cranial fossa containing the temporal lobes of the brain and the hypophysis cerebri (pituitary gland).
3 – Posterior cranial fossa containing cerebellum, pons and medulla oblongata.

ORBITAL CAVITY (Fig. 10.4)

Bones forming the orbital cavity

Sphenoid bone – the greater and lesser wings.

Zygomatic bone – orbital surface and border.

Ethmoid bone – orbital plate.

Palatine bone – orbital process.

Frontal bone – supraorbital margin and the orbital plate.

Lacrimal bone – orbital surface.

Maxilla – orbital surface.

Features of the orbital cavity

The orbital cavity contains the eyeball, its muscles, nerves and blood vessels, and the lacrimal gland.

Superior orbital fissure – transmits the oculomotor, trochlear and abducent nerves, ophthalmic division of the trigeminal nerve and the ophthalmic veins.

Inferior orbital fissure – transmits the maxillary nerve.

Supraorbital foramen (notch) – transmits the supraorbital vessels and nerves.

Optic foramen – opening of the optic canal.

Optic canal – transmits the optic nerve and the ophthalmic artery.

Infraorbital groove – contains the infraorbital nerve before it passes through the infraorbital canal to the infraorbital foramen.

Lacrimal groove – in which the lacrimal sac is situated.

Nasolacrimal canal – carries the nasolacrimal duct from the lacrimal gland to the nasal cavity.

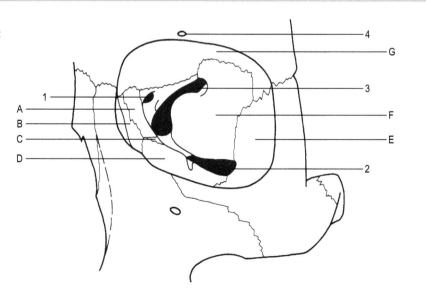

Fig. 10.4 Bones forming the left orbit (anterior aspect).
A – Ethmoid bone
B – Lacrimal bone
C – Palatine bone
D – Maxilla
E – Zygomatic bone
F – Sphenoid bone
G – Frontal bone.

Structures associated with the left orbit – anterior aspect
1 – Optic canal (foramen)
2 – Inferior orbital fissure
3 – Superior orbital fissure
4 – Supraorbital foramen (notch).

Radiographic appearances of the orbital cavity (Figs 10.5 and 10.6)

Fig. 10.5 Optic foramen: right oblique projection. (From Bryan 1996.)
A – Supraorbital margin
B – Optic foramen
C – Petrous temporal bone
D – Petrous temporal bone
E – Posterior ethmoidal sinuses
F – Lesser wing of sphenoid
G – Frontal sinus.

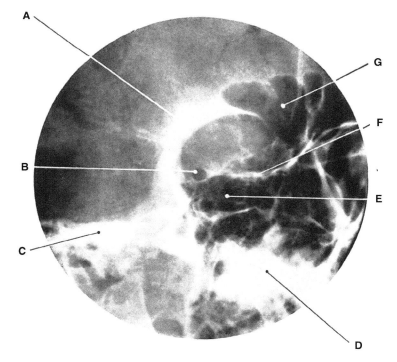

Fig. 10.6 CT scan through orbits. (From Bryan 1996.)
1 – Pterygoid
2 – Sphenoid bone
3 – Medial rectus muscle
4 – Optic nerve
5 – Lateral rectus muscle
6 – Globe
7 – Lens.

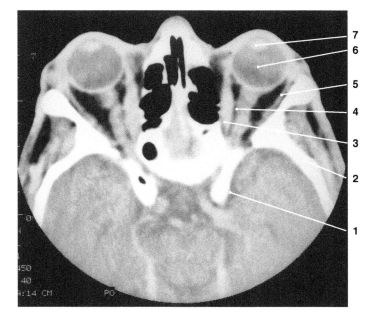

NASAL CAVITY (Fig. 10.7)

Forms the upper part of the respiratory tract and is irregular in shape.

Roof

Formed by:
Nasal septum of the frontal and nasal bones.
Cribriform plate of the ethmoid bone.
Body of the sphenoid bone.

Floor

Forms the division between the oral and nasal cavities. Formed by:
Palatine process of the maxilla.
Horizontal plate of the palatine bone.

Medial wall

Referred to as the nasal septum. Formed by:
Vomer.
Perpendicular plate of the ethmoid bone.
Septal cartilage.

Lateral wall

Irregular as it forms the 3 nasal conchae. Formed by:
Nasal surface of the maxilla.
Perpendicular plate of the palatine bone.
Ethmoidal labyrinth.
Inferior nasal concha.

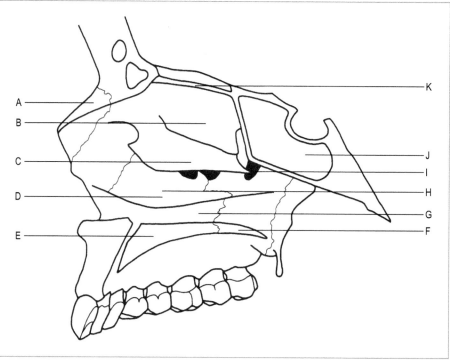

Fig. 10.7 Nasal cavity (sagittal section).
A – Nasal bone
B – Superior concha
C – Middle concha
D – Inferior concha
E – Maxilla
F – Horizontal plate of the palatine bone
G – Inferior meatus
H – Middle meatus
I – Spheno-ethmoidal recess
J – Sphenoidal sinus
K – Cribriform plate of the ethmoid bone.

Conchae	*Superior nasal concha* – projection from the ethmoid bone.
	Middle nasal concha – part of the ethmoid bone.
	Inferior nasal concha – a separate bone.

Spheno-ethmoidal recess
Above and behind the superior concha.
Communicates with the sphenoidal sinus.

Superior meatus
Forms attachment for the superior nasal concha.
Communicates with the posterior ethmoidal sinuses.

Middle meatus
Lies between the middle and inferior nasal conchae.
Communicates with the anterior ethmoidal sinuses, the middle ethmoidal sinuses, the frontal sinus and the maxillary sinus.

Inferior meatus
Lies below the inferior nasal concha.
Communicates with the orbit via the nasolacrimal canal.

PARANASAL SINUSES (Figs 10.8 and 10.9)

Consist of:

    Maxillary sinuses (2)
    Frontal sinuses (2)
    Ethmoidal sinuses (3 groups)
    Sphenoidal sinuses (2).

The sinuses are lined with mucous membrane, which is continuous with that of the nasal cavity.

Function	To lighten the skull.
	To add resonance to the voice.

Maxillary sinuses (largest) (Fig. 10.8)

Shape	Pyramidal cavities.
Position	They lie on either side of the nasal cavity, below the orbits.
Structure	*Base* – formed by the lateral wall of the nasal cavity.
	Apex – projects into the zygomatic process of the maxilla.

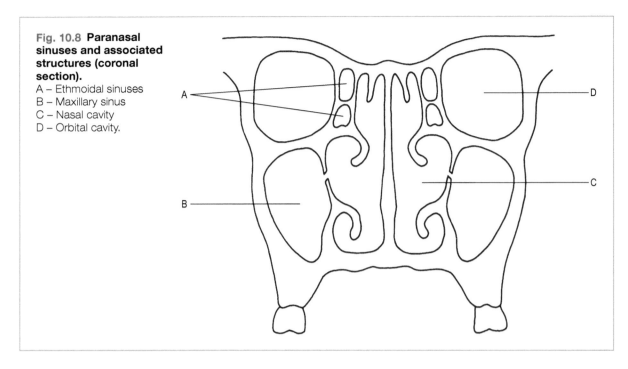

Fig. 10.8 Paranasal sinuses and associated structures (coronal section).
A – Ethmoidal sinuses
B – Maxillary sinus
C – Nasal cavity
D – Orbital cavity.

Floor – formed by the alveolar process of the maxilla.

Roof – formed by the floor of the orbit.

Communication (Fig. 10.9) — With the middle meatus of the nasal cavity via the antral ostium.

Frontal sinuses (Fig. 10.8)

Shape — Irregular.

Position — In the midline above the nasal cavity and the orbits, in front of the anterior cranial fossa, behind the superciliary arches.

Structure — Vary in size and shape from person to person. Are divided from each other by a septum, near the midline.

Communication (Fig. 10.9) — With the middle meatus of the nose via the frontonasal canal or ethmoidal infundibulum.

Ethmoidal sinuses (Fig. 10.8)

Shape — Numerous small cavities, irregular in shape.

Position — Situated between the medial wall of the orbit and the nasal cavity, in the ethmoidal labyrinth, below the anterior cranial fossa.

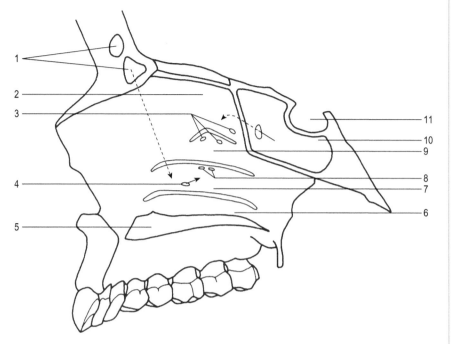

Fig. 10.9 Paranasal sinuses and associated structures (sagittal section).
1 – Frontal sinuses
2 – Spheno-ethmoidal recess
3 – Opening for the ethmoidal sinuses
4 – Opening for the maxillary sinuses
5 – Hard palate
6 – Inferior meatus
7 – Middle meatus
8 – Opening for ethmoidal sinuses
9 – Superior meatus
10 – Sphenoidal sinuses
11 – Sella turcica (hypophyseal fossa, pituitary fossa).

Structure	Divided into 3 groups: anterior, middle and posterior.
	Orbital plate – forms the boundary between the sinus and the medial wall of the orbit.
	Medial plate – forms the boundary between the sinus and the lateral wall of the nasal cavity.
Communication (Fig. 10.9)	*Anterior and middle groups* – via the spheno-ethmoidal recess above the superior conchae of the nasal cavity.
	Posterior group – with the superior meatus of the nasal cavity.

Sphenoidal sinuses (Fig. 10.9)

Shape	Cuboidal.
Position	In the body of the sphenoid bone below the sella turcica, hypophysis cerebri (pituitary gland) and the hypothalamus of the brain, above and behind the nasal cavity and the ethmoidal sinuses.
Communication (Fig. 10.9)	With the spheno-ethmoidal recess in the nasal cavity.

Radiographic appearances of the paranasal sinuses (Figs 10.10 to 10.18)

Fig. 10.10 Nasal sinuses: occipito-mental projection.
(From Bryan 1996.)
1 – Orbit
2 – Nasal septum
3 – Maxillary antrium
4 – Zygoma
5 – Sphenoid sinus
6 – Infraorbital foramen
7 – Ethmoid air cells
8 – Frontal sinus.

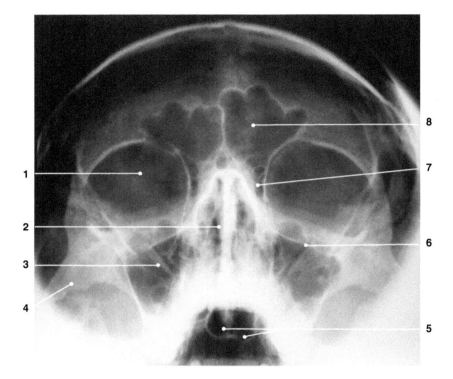

Fig. 10.11 Radio-graphic projection of the nasal sinuses: occipitomental.
(From Bryan 1996.)
F – Frontal sinus
R – Right orbit
L – Left orbit
M – Maxillary sinus
S – Sphenoid sinuses.

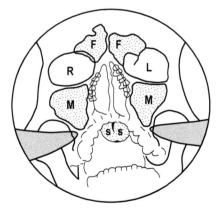

INSIGHT

Fluid can collect in the maxillary antrum, this will not be demonstrated unless a horizontal beam is used. Any angulation of the beam could give the appearance of thickening of the lining of the antrum rather than fluid.

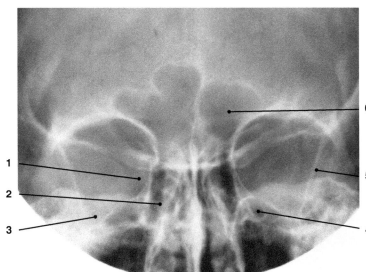

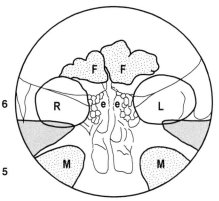

Fig. 10.12 Nasal sinuses: occipitofrontal projection.
(From Bryan 1996.)

1 – Superior orbital fissure
2 – Ethmoid air cells
3 – Petrous temporal bone
4 – Foramen rotundum
5 – Innominate line
6 – Frontal sinus.

Fig. 10.13 Radiographic projection of the nasal sinuses: 20° occipitofrontal. (From Bryan 1996.)
F – Frontal sinus
e – Ethmoidal sinuses
R – Right orbit
L – Left orbit
M – Maxillary sinus

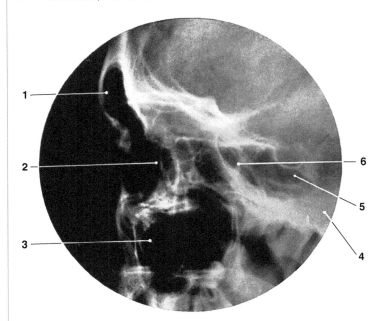

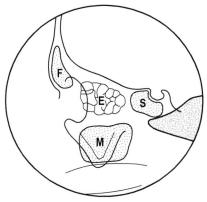

Fig. 10.15 Radiographic projection of the nasal sinuses: lateral. (From Bryan 1996.)
F – Frontal sinus
E – Ethmoidal sinuses
M – Maxillary sinus
S – Sphenoidal sinuses.

Fig. 10.14 Nasal sinuses: lateral projection. (From Bryan 1996.)

1 – Frontal sinuses
2 – Anterior margin of ethmoidal sinuses
3 – Maxillary sinuses
4 – Petrous temporal bones
5 – Sphenoidal sinuses
6 – Posterior margin of ethmoidal sinuses.

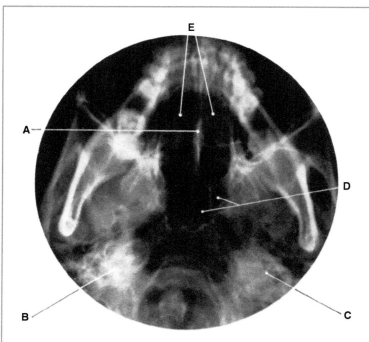

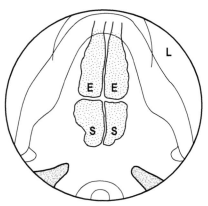

Fig. 10.17 Radiographic projection of the nasal sinuses: submentovertical. (From Bryan 1996.)
E – Ethmoidal sinuses
S – Sphenoidal sinus sinuses.
L – Left (Normal radiographic label).

Fig. 10.16 Nasal sinuses: submentovertical projection.
(From Bryan 1996.)

A – Nasal septum
B – Petrous temporal bone
C – Petrous temporal bone
D – Sphenoidal sinuses
E – Posterior ethmoidal sinuses.

Fig. 10.18 Sinuses: CT scan.
A – Maxillary sinus
B – Inferior concha
C – Middle concha
D – Posterior ethmoid air cells
E – Orbit and contents
F – Nasal septum.

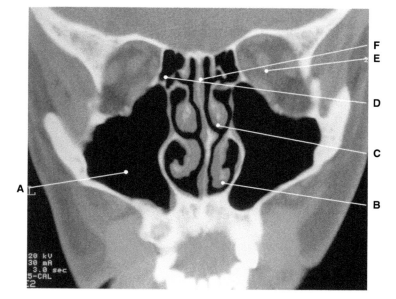

FEATURES OF THE SKULL (Figs 10.19 to 10.23)

Fig. 10.19 Foramina in the base of the skull (internal aspect).

A – Optic canal, for the optic nerve and the ophthalmic artery.

B – Foramen rotundum, for the maxillary division of the trigeminal nerve.

C – Foramen ovale, for the mandibular division of the trigeminal nerve.

D – Foramen spinosum, for the middle meningeal artery.

E – Foramen magnum, for part of the medulla oblongata, the spinal roots of accessory nerves and the vertebral arteries.

F – Hypoglossal canal, for the hypoglossal nerve and the meningeal branch of the ascending pharyngeal artery.

G – Jugular foramen, for the internal jugular vein, the glossopharyngeal, vagus and accessory nerves and the inferior petrosal sinus.

H – Internal acoustic (auditory) meatus, for the facial and auditory nerves.

I – Foramen lacerum. The lower part is closed by fibrocartilage; the internal carotid artery crosses it (after entering by the carotid canal).

J – Cribriform plate, for the olfactory nerve filaments.

Carotid canal – lies on the external aspect, for the internal carotid artery.

Stylomastoid foramen – lies on the external aspect between the styloid and mastoid processes of the temporal bone, for the facial nerve.

Superior orbital fissure – concealed by the lesser wing of the sphenoid bone, for the oculomotor, trochlear and abducent nerves, ophthalmic division of the trigeminal nerve and the ophthalmic veins.

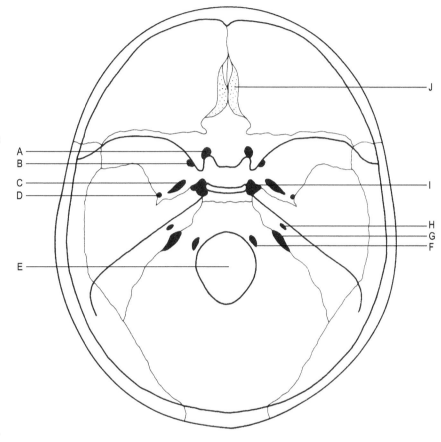

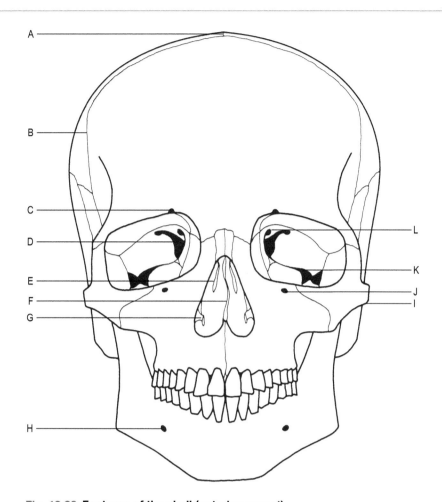

Fig. 10.20 Features of the skull (anterior aspect).
A – Sagittal suture
B – Coronal suture
C – Supraorbital notch (foramen)
D – Superior orbital fissure
E – Middle nasal concha
F – Vomer
G – Inferior nasal concha
H – Mental foramen
I – Zygomatic arch
J – Infraorbital foramen
K – Inferior orbital fissure
L – Optic canal.

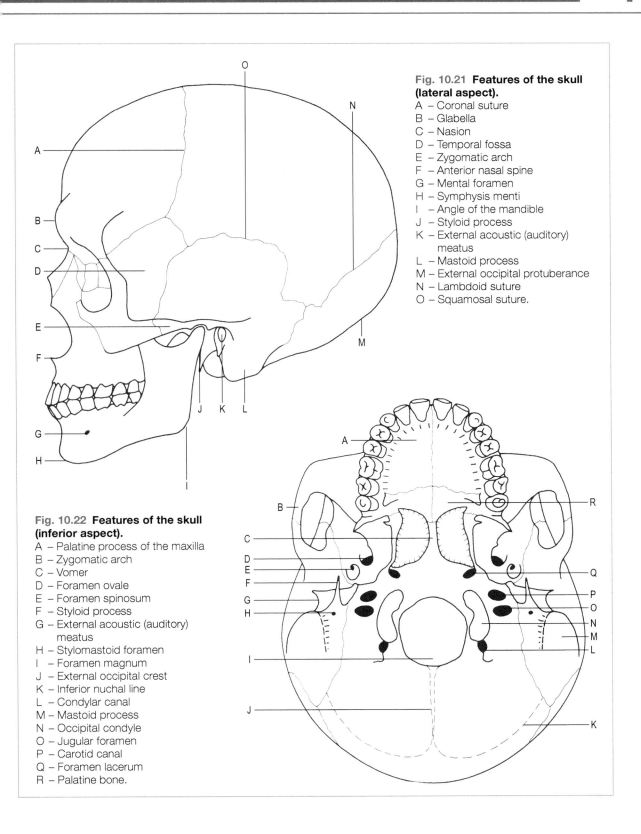

Fig. 10.21 Features of the skull (lateral aspect).
A – Coronal suture
B – Glabella
C – Nasion
D – Temporal fossa
E – Zygomatic arch
F – Anterior nasal spine
G – Mental foramen
H – Symphysis menti
I – Angle of the mandible
J – Styloid process
K – External acoustic (auditory) meatus
L – Mastoid process
M – External occipital protuberance
N – Lambdoid suture
O – Squamosal suture.

Fig. 10.22 Features of the skull (inferior aspect).
A – Palatine process of the maxilla
B – Zygomatic arch
C – Vomer
D – Foramen ovale
E – Foramen spinosum
F – Styloid process
G – External acoustic (auditory) meatus
H – Stylomastoid foramen
I – Foramen magnum
J – External occipital crest
K – Inferior nuchal line
L – Condylar canal
M – Mastoid process
N – Occipital condyle
O – Jugular foramen
P – Carotid canal
Q – Foramen lacerum
R – Palatine bone.

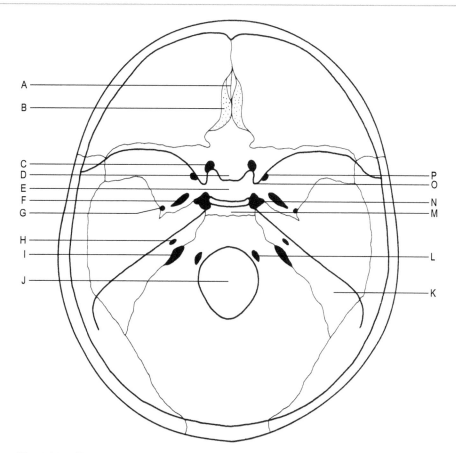

Fig. 10.23 Features of the skull (cranial cavity).
A – Crista galli of the ethmoid bone
B – Cribriform plate of the ethmoid bone
C – Optic foramen
D – Tuberculum sellae of the sphenoid bone
E – Sella turcica (hypophyseal fossa, pituitary fossa) of the sphenoid bone
F – Foramen ovale
G – Foramen spinosum
H – Internal acoustic (auditory) meatus
I – Jugular foramen
J – Foramen magnum
K – Petrous portion of the temporal bone
L – Hypoglossal canal
M – Dorsum sellae
N – Foramen lacerum
O – Anterior clinoid process of the sphenoid bone
P – Foramen rotundum.

Radiographic appearances of the skull (Figs 10.24 to 10.30)

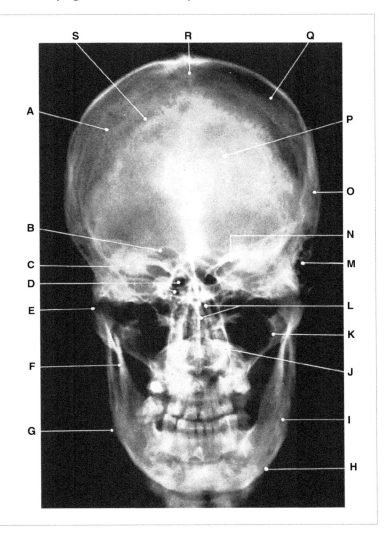

Fig. 10.24 Cranial bones: occipitofrontal projection.
(From Bryan 1996.)

A – Coronal suture
B – Frontal sinus
C – Petrous part of temporal bone
D – Ethmoidal sinuses
E – Head of mandible
F – Coronoid process
G – Angle of mandible
H – Body of mandible
I – Mandibular canal
J – Inferior nasal concha
K – Maxillary sinus
L – Ethmoid bone in nasal cavity
M – Mastoid air cells
N – Supraorbital margin
O – Squamous part of temporal bone
P – Frontal bone
Q – Parietal bone
R – Sagittal suture
S – Lambdoid suture.

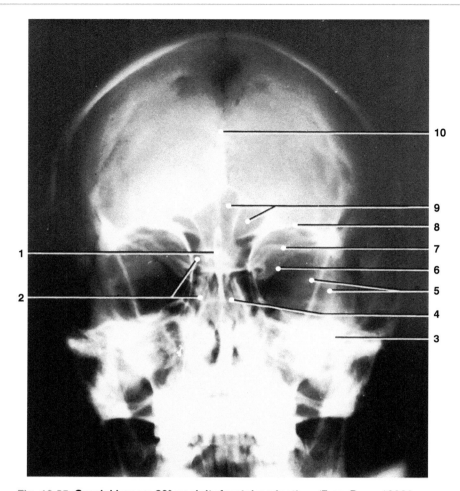

Fig. 10.25 Cranial bones: 20° occipitofrontal projection. (From Bryan 1996.)

1 – Crista galli
2 – Ethmoid air cells
3 – Mastoid air cells
4 – Floor of pituitary fossa
5 – Greater wing of sphenoid
6 – Superior orbital fissure
7 – Lesser wing of sphenoid
8 – Supraorbital margin
9 – Frontal sinus
10 – Sagittal suture.

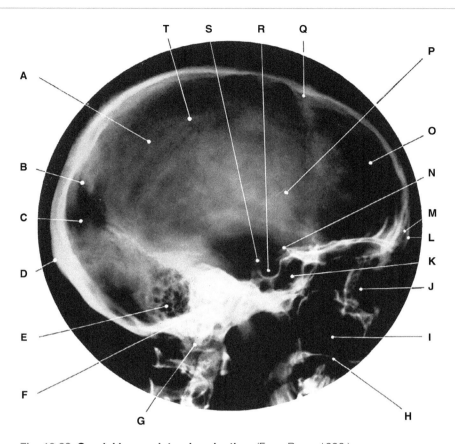

Fig. 10.26 Cranial bones: lateral projection. (From Bryan 1996.)

A – Parietal bones
B – Lambdoid suture
C – Occipital bone
D – External occipital protuberance
E – Mastoid air cells
F – Petrous part of temporal bones
G – Mastoid process
H – Hard palate
I – Maxillary sinuses
J – Orbital cavities
K – Sphenoidal sinuses
L – Glabella
M – Frontal sinuses
N – Anterior clinoid processes
O – Frontal bone
P – Groove for middle meningeal artery
Q – Coronal suture
R – Sella turcica
S – Dorsum sellae
T – Channels of diploic vein.

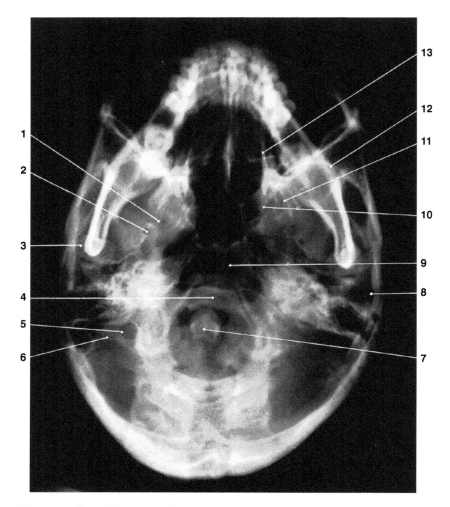

Fig. 10.27 Cranial bones: submentovertical projection. (From Bryan 1996.)

1 – Foramen ovale
2 – Foramen spinosum
3 – Head of mandible
4 – Anterior arch of atlas
5 – Foramen transversarium
6 – Transverse process of atlas
7 – Odontoid process
8 – External auditory meatus
9 – Pharynx
10 – Medial pterygoid plate
11 – Lateral pterygoid plate
12 – Anterior wall of middle cranial fossa
13 – Lateral wall of nasal cavity.

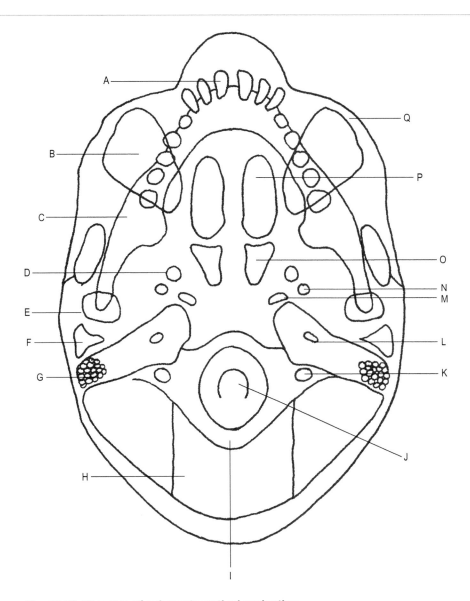

Fig. 10.28 Diagram of submentovertical projection.

A – Incisor tooth
B – Maxillary sinus
C – Angle of mandible
D – Foramen ovale
E – Head of mandible
F – External auditory meatus
G – Mastoid air cells
H – Cervical spine
I – Posterior arch of atlas

J – Odontoid process
K – Foramen transversarium
L – Internal auditory meatus
M – Foramen lacerum
N – Foramen spinosum
O – Sphenoid sinus
P – Ethmoid sinus
Q – Zygomatic arch.

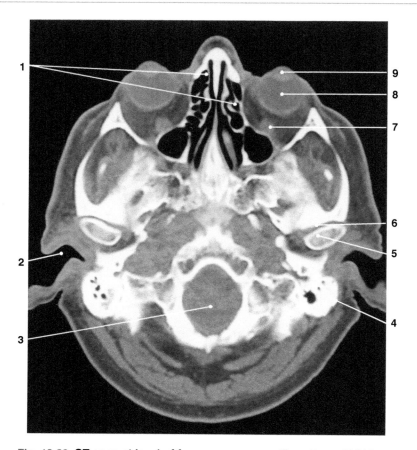

Fig. 10.29 CT scan at level of foramen magnum. (From Bryan 1996.)

1 – Ethmoid air cells
2 – External auditory meatus
3 – Foramen magnum
4 – Petrous bone
5 – Condyle of mandible
6 – Temporomandibular joint
7 – Superior rectus muscle
8 – Globe
9 – Lens.

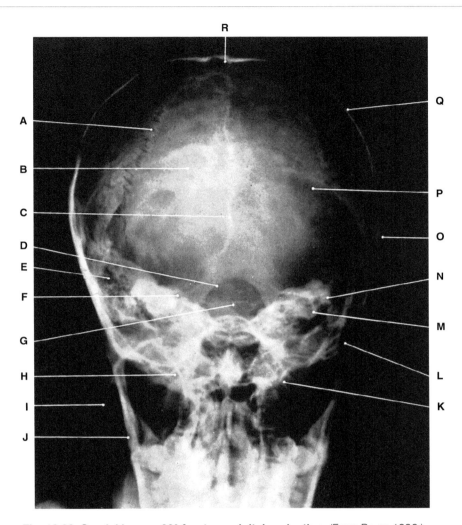

Fig. 10.30 Cranial bones: 30° fronto-occipital projection. (From Bryan 1996.)

A – Lambdoid suture
B – Occipital bone
C – Occipital crest
D – Foramen magnum
E – Mastoid air cells
F – Internal auditory meatus
G – Dorsum sellae
H – Inferior orbital fissure
I – Zygomatic arch
J – Ramus of mandible

K – Roof of maxillary sinus
L – Mastoid process
M – Cochlea
N – Semicircular canals
O – Temporal bone
P – Transverse sulcus
Q – Parietal bone
R – Sagittal suture.

INDIVIDUAL BONES OF THE SKULL

Occipital bone (Fig. 10.31)

Type	Flat bone.
Position	Forms the posterior part of the base of the skull.
Articulations	*The occipital condyles* with the 1st cervical vertebra to form the atlanto-occipital joint.
	The squamous part with the temporal bone and the parietal bones to form the lambdoid suture.
Main parts	The bone can be divided into 3 areas:

Squamous part
This lies posterior to the foramen magnum.

Internal surface – concave, divided into 4 fossae by:

- *horizontal groove* – for the transverse venous sinus; the tentorium cerebelli is attached to the edge of the groove.
- *sulcus for superior sagittal venous sinus* – situated above the horizontal groove; the margins provide attachment for the falx cerebri
- *internal occipital crest* – below the horizontal groove.

Internal occipital protuberance – where the vertical grooves meet.

External surface – convex.

External occipital crest – midline structure from the foramen magnum to the external occipital protuberance.

External occipital protuberance – midway between the foramen magnum and the superior aspect of the bone.

Superior nuchal lines – run-laterally from the external occipital protuberance.

Highest nuchal lines – faint lines above the superior nuchal lines.

Inferior nuchal lines – below the superior nuchal lines, running laterally from the external occipital crest.

Basilar part
This lies anterior to the foramen magnum.

Pharyngeal tubercle – lies on the inferior surface, 1 cm anterior to the foramen magnum, in the midline; provides attachment for the pharynx.

Clivus – lies on the superior surface; runs upwards and forwards from the anterior border of the foramen magnum; forms attachment for the membrana tectoria and the apical ligament.

Lateral (condylar) parts
These lie on either side of the foramen magnum.

Occipital condyles – lie on the inferior surface, on either side of the foramen magnum, and articulate with the atlas.

Fig. 10.31 Occipital bone (external surface).
A – Squamous part
B – Highest nuchal line
C – External occipital protuberance
D – Superior nuchal line
E – Inferior nuchal line
F – External occipital crest
G – Condylar canal
H – Jugular process
I – Condyle
J – Basilar part
K – Hypoglossal canal
L – Jugular notch
M – Condylar fossa
N – Foramen magnum.

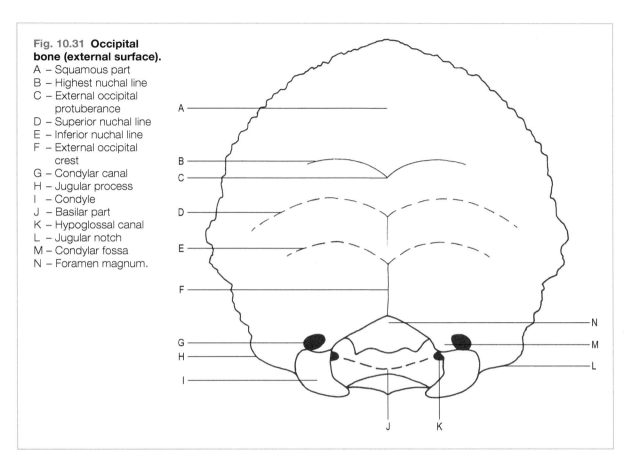

Hypoglossal canal – situated above the condyles, on the rim of the foramen magnum; carries the hypoglossal nerve and the meningeal branch of the ascending pharyngeal artery.

Condylar fossa – lies posterior to the condyle; receives the superior facet of the atlas when the head is extended.

Jugular process – lateral to the condyle.

Jugular notch – on the jugular process, forms the posterior aspect of the jugular foramen.

Jugular tubercle – on the superior surface, above the hypoglossal canal.

Foramen magnum – large foramen for part of the medulla oblongata, the accessory nerves and the vertebral arteries.

Ossification

Primary centres

Squamous part – 4 centres.

Lateral parts – 2 centres.

Basilar part – 1 centre.

Sphenoid bone (Figs 10.32 and 10.33)

Type	Irregular bone.
Position	Forms part of the base of the skull, lying between the frontal, temporal and occipital bones.
Articulations	*The greater wings* with the temporal bone to form the sphenosquamosal suture. With the *vomer, ethmoid, occipital, frontal, zygomatic* and *palatine* bones.
Main parts	The bone consists of a body, 2 pairs of wings and 2 pterygoid processes.

Body

Superior surface – articulates with the ethmoid bone.

Optic canal (foramen) – lateral part of the superior surface for the optic nerve.

Tuberculum sellae – posterior to the optic canals, forming the anterior boundary of the sella turcica.

Sella turcica – posterior to the tuberculum sellae; contains the hypophysis cerebri (pituitary gland).

Middle clinoid processes – lateral projections on the tuberculum sellae.

Anterior clinoid processes – lateral to the middle clinoid processes.

Dorsum sellae – posterior part of the sella turcica.

Clivus – posterior to the dorsum sellae and articulates with the clivus of the occipital bone.

Lateral surfaces – junction of the body and greater wings.

Carotid sulcus – above the lateral surfaces; carries the internal carotid artery and the cavernous venous sinus.

Anterior surface – articulates with the ethmoid bone.

Sphenoidal crest – on the anterior surface; forms part of the nasal septum.

Sphenoidal sinus – in the body, see paranasal sinuses, pp. 207–210.

Sphenoidal conchae – 2 thin plates on the anterior aspect of the body.

Inferior surface – has several processes:

- *sphenoidal rostrum* – process in the midline; forms articulation with the vomer
- *vaginal processes* – processes on either side of rostrum.

Greater wings

Two processes from the sides of the body.

Sphenosquamosal suture – junction between the greater wings and the squamous part of the temporal bone.

Cerebral surface – forms part of the middle cranial fossa; presents with 3 foramina:

- *foramen rotundum* – on the antero-medial surface, for the maxillary nerve
- *foramen ovale* – postero-lateral to the foramen rotundum, for the mandibular nerve and the accessory meningeal artery.

Fig. 10.32 Sphenoid bone (anterior aspect).
A – Lesser wing
B – Superior orbital fissure
C – Sphenoidal crest
D – Foramen rotundum
E – Foramen ovale
F – Vaginal process
G – Lateral pterygoid plate
H – Pterygoid hamulus
I – Sphenoidal rostrum
J – Medial pterygoid plate
K – Spine
L – Orbital surface
M – Temporal surface.

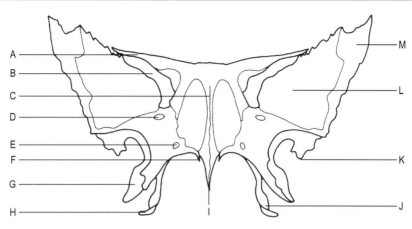

Fig. 10.33 Sphenoid bone (superior aspect).
1 – Greater wing
2 – Lesser wing
3 – Optic canal (foramen)
4 – Superior orbital fissure
5 – Anterior clinoid process
6 – Foramen rotundum
7 – Foramen ovale
8 – Foramen spinosum
9 – Posterior clinoid process
10 – Dorsum sellae
11 – Spine
12 – Sella turcica
13 – Tuberculum sellae
14 – Ethmoidal spine.

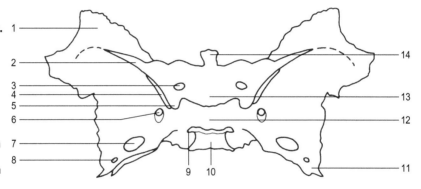

■ *foramen spinosum* – medial to the foramen ovale, for the middle meningeal artery and the meningeal branch of the mandibular nerve.

Orbital surface – forms the posterior part of the lateral wall of the orbit.

Postero-lateral border of inferior orbital fissure – formed by the inferior border of the orbital surface.

Lateral border of superior orbital fissure – formed by the medial border of the orbital surface.

Anterior border of foramen lacerum – formed by the posterior border of the junction of the greater wing with the body.

Lesser wings
Lesser wings – triangular plates projecting laterally from upper surface of the body.

Superior surfaces – support part of frontal lobe of the cerebrum.

Inferior surfaces – form part of roof of orbit.

Upper border of superior orbital fissure – formed by inferior surface of the lesser wings.

Optic canal – at the junction of the lesser wings and the body.

Superior orbital fissure – carries the oculomotor, trochlear and abducent nerves, and branches of the trigeminal nerves and middle meningeal artery.

Pterygoid processes
Pterygoid processes project downwards from the junction of the greater wings and body.

Lateral pterygoid plate – flat plate of bone.

Medial pterygoid plate – narrow and long, medial to the lateral pterygoid plate.

Pterygoid hamulus – hook-shaped process on the end of the medial pterygoid plate.

Pterygoid fissure – at the junction between the 2 plates.

Ossification	*Anterior aspect of the bone* – 6 centres.
	Posterior aspect of the bone – 8 centres.

Temporal bone (Figs 10.34 and 10.35)

Type	Irregular bones.
Position	Form the side and part of the base of the skull.
Articulations	*Mandibular fossa* with the head of mandible to form the temporomandibular joint.
	The squamous part with the parietal bones to form the squamosal suture and with the occipital bones to form the lambdoid suture.
	With the greater wings of sphenoid to form the sphenosquamosal suture.
	With the zygomatic bone.
Main parts	The bone is formed by 3 parts:

Squamous part
Forms the upper anterior part of the bone.

Temporal surface – forms part of the temporal fossa.

Zygoma – articulates with the zygomatic bone and forms the mandibular fossa.

Mandibular fossa – articulates with the articular disc of the temporomandibular joint. Its posterior aspect is non-articular.

Petromastoid part
This is formed by a mastoid and a petrous part.

Fig. 10.34 Left temporal bone (external aspect).
A – Squamous part
B – Zygoma
C – Mandibular fossa
D – External acoustic (auditory) meatus
E – Tympanic plate
F – Styloid process
G – Mastoid process
H – Mastoid part.

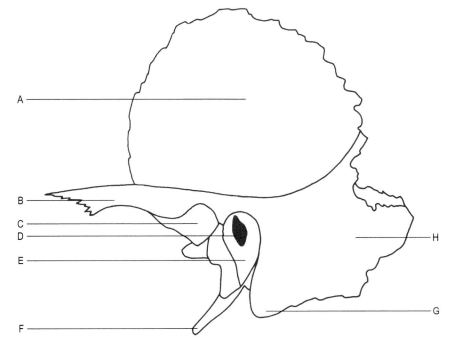

Fig. 10.35 Left temporal bone (posterior aspect).
1 – Squamous part
2 – Zygomatic process
3 – Mastoid process
4 – Mastoid notch
5 – Styloid process
6 – Petrous part
7 – Internal acoustic (auditory) meatus.

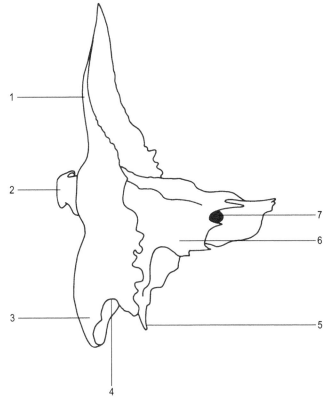

Mastoid part – forms posterior aspect of the bone:

mastoid process – contains the mastoid air cells, which vary in size from person to person

mastoid notch – on the medial aspect of the mastoid process.

Petrous part – lies between the sphenoid and occipital bones in the base of the skull:

apex – forms the postero-lateral boundary of the foramen lacerum.

anterior surface – forms part of the floor of the middle cranial fossa.

posterior surface – forms the anterior aspect of the posterior cranial cavity.

internal acoustic (auditory) meatus – lies on the posterior surface of the petrous part and carries the facial and auditory nerves.

carotid canal – lies on the inferior surface of the petrous part and carries the internal carotid artery.

jugular fossa – lies behind the opening of the carotid canal; with the jugular notch of the occipital bone forms the jugular foramen which carries the internal jugular vein and the glossopharyngeal, vagus and accessory nerves.

Tympanic part

This lies in front of the mastoid process.

External acoustic (auditory) meatus – mainly lies in the tympanic part; extends to the tympanic membrane, which forms the boundary of the middle ear.

Stylomastoid foramen – between the mastoid and styloid processes and carries the stylomastoid artery and the facial nerve.

Styloid process – lies anterior to the mastoid process and forms attachment for the stylohyoid ligament.

Middle ear

Lies between the external acoustic meatus and the inner ear; contains the auditory ossicles:

Malleus – hammer-shaped; is in contact with the tympanic membrane.

Incus – anvil-shaped; lies between the malleus and the stapes.

Stapes – stirrup-shaped; lies at the junction of the middle and inner ear.

Inner ear

Medial to the middle ear in the petrous part of the temporal bone.

Bony labyrinth – contains the organs of hearing and balance.

Vestibule – central part of the cavity, roughly oval in shape.

Semicircular canals – 3 canals: superior, posterior and lateral; lie postero-superior to the vestibule.

Cochlea – snail-shell-shaped; lies anterior to the vestibule.

Ossification

Squamous part – 1 centre.

Petromastoid part – up to 14 centres.

Tympanic part – 1 centre.

Styloid process – 2 centres.

Radiographic appearances of the temporal bone (Figs 10.36, 10.37 and 10.38)

Fig. 10.36 Temporal bone: lateral oblique projection.
(From Bryan 1996.)
A – Mastoid antrum
B – Edge of sigmoid sulcus
C – Mastoid process
D – Jugular foramen
E – Posterior border of ramus of mandible
F – Head of mandible
G – Zygomatic arch
H – External auditory meatus
I – Tegmen tympani.

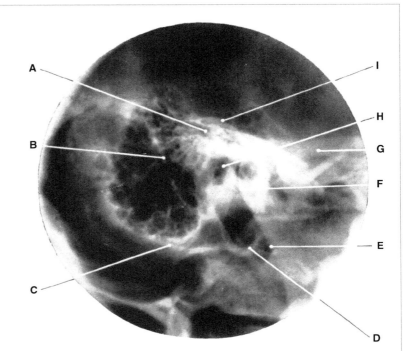

Fig. 10.37 Temporal bone: modified Stenver's projection.
(From Bryan 1996.)
1 – Internal auditory canal
2 – Cochlea
3 – Vestibule
4 – Lateral semicircular canal
5 – Arcuate eminence
6 – Superior semicircular canal.

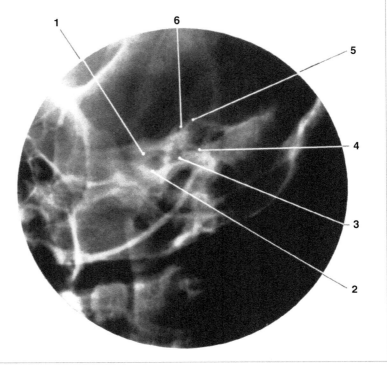

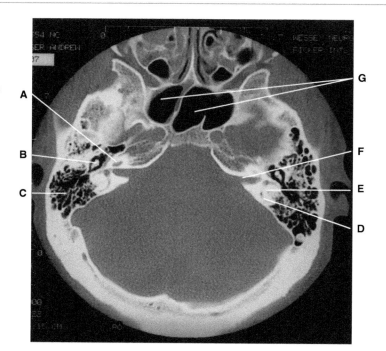

Fig. 10.38 CT scan through middle and internal ear. (From Bryan 1996.)
A – Cochlea
B – Malleus and incus
C – Mastoid air cells
D – Posterior semicircular canal
E – Horizontal semicircular canal
F – Internal auditory canal
G – Sphenoid sinus.

Parietal bones (Fig. 10.39)

Type	Irregular bones.
Position	Form the sides and the roof of the cranium.
Articulations	*With the sagittal border* of the opposite parietal bone to form the sagittal suture. *With the frontal bone* to form part of the coronal suture. *With the occipital bone* to form part of the lambdoid suture. *With the sphenoid and temporal bones.*
Main parts	Each bone has 2 surfaces, 4 borders and 4 angles. *External surface* – convex, and has 2 curved lines, the superior and inferior temporal lines. *Internal surface* – concave, and has a groove for the superior sagittal sinus and some depressions (granular foveolae) for the arachnoid granulations. *Sagittal border* – on the superior aspect. *Squamosal border* – on the inferior aspect; articulates with the sphenoid and temporal bones. *Frontal border* – on the anterior aspect.

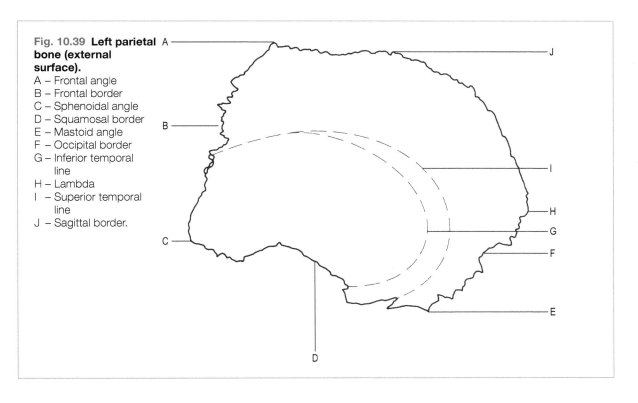

Fig. 10.39 Left parietal bone (external surface).
A – Frontal angle
B – Frontal border
C – Sphenoidal angle
D – Squamosal border
E – Mastoid angle
F – Occipital border
G – Inferior temporal line
H – Lambda
I – Superior temporal line
J – Sagittal border.

Occipital border – on the posterior aspect.

Sphenoidal angle – at the junction of the squamosal and frontal borders; has a groove for the frontal branch of the middle meningeal vessels.

Occipital angle – at the junction of the occipital and sagittal borders (and therefore at the junction of the sagittal and lambdoid sutures, which is called the lambda).

Mastoid angle – at the junction of the occipital and squamosal borders.

Frontal angle – at the junction of the sagittal and frontal borders (and therefore at the junction of the sagittal and coronal sutures, which is called the bregma).

| *Ossification* | *2* primary centres. |

Frontal bone (Figs 10.40 and 10.41)

Type	Flat bone.
Position	Forms the front of the cranium, above the orbits.
Articulations	With the *maxillae, zygomatic, nasal, lacrimal, ethmoid* and *sphenoid* bones.
Main parts	*External surface* – convex.
	Supraorbital margins – form the upper border of the orbits.

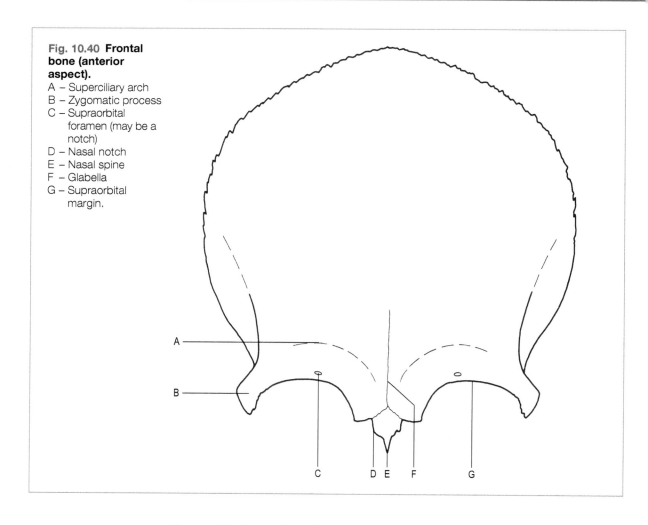

Fig. 10.40 Frontal bone (anterior aspect).
A – Superciliary arch
B – Zygomatic process
C – Supraorbital foramen (may be a notch)
D – Nasal notch
E – Nasal spine
F – Glabella
G – Supraorbital margin.

Supraorbital notch – for the supraorbital vessels and nerves; may be a foramen.

Zygomatic process – lateral end of the supraorbital margin; articulates with the zygomatic bone.

Nasal part – between supraorbital margins.

Nasal spine – forms the end of the nasal part; forms part of the nasal septum.

Nasal notches – either side of the nasal spine; articulate with the nasal bones.

Superciliary arches – above the supraorbital margins.

Glabella – junction of the 2 superciliary arches.

Internal surface – concave.

Vertical groove – in the midline for the sagittal venous sinus.

Frontal crest – edges of vertical groove for attachment for the falx cerebri.

Granular foveolae – indentations for the arachnoid granulations.

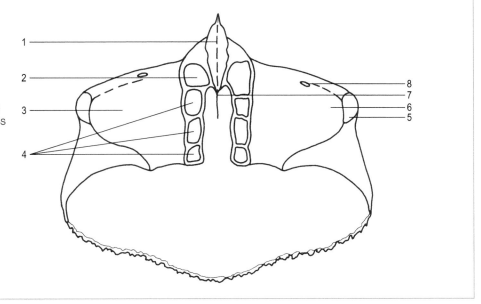

Fig. 10.41 Frontal bone (inferior aspect).
1 – Nasal spine
2 – Frontal sinus
3 – Orbital plate
4 – Roofs of the ethmoidal sinuses
5 – Zygomatic process
6 – Fossa for the lacrimal gland
7 – Frontal crest
8 – Supraorbital foramen (may be a notch).

Parietal margin – articulates with the greater wing of the sphenoid bone.

Orbital plates – concave; form the roof of the orbit.

Fossa for lacrimal gland – antero-lateral aspect of the orbital plates.

Ethmoidal notch – at the junction of the orbital plates; occupied by the cribriform plate of the ethmoid bone.

Frontal sinuses – see paranasal sinuses, pp. 206–210.

Ossification   2 primary centres.

Ethmoid bone (Fig. 10.42)

Type   Irregular bone.

Position   Behind the nasal bones, between the orbits.

Articulations   With the *vomer, maxillae,* and the *frontal, palatine, lacrimal* and *sphenoid* bones.

Main parts   The bone is formed by 2 plates and 2 labyrinths.

Cribriform plate
Lies in the ethmoid notch of the frontal bone and forms the roof of the nasal cavity.

Crista galli – in the midline of the cribriform plate; forms attachment for the falx cerebri.

Foramina – in the cribriform plate for the olfactory nerve filaments.

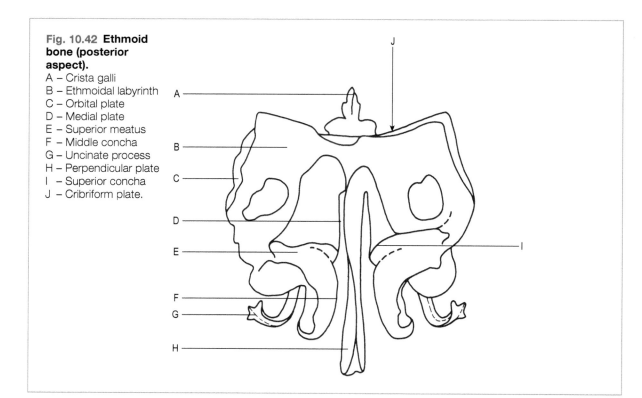

Fig. 10.42 Ethmoid bone (posterior aspect).
A – Crista galli
B – Ethmoidal labyrinth
C – Orbital plate
D – Medial plate
E – Superior meatus
F – Middle concha
G – Uncinate process
H – Perpendicular plate
I – Superior concha
J – Cribriform plate.

Perpendicular plate
In the midline of the cribriform plate; forms part of the nasal septum.

Ethmoidal labyrinths
Lie at either side of the perpendicular plate.
Ethmoidal air cells – see the paranasal sinuses, pp. 206–210.
Orbital plate – forms medial wall of the orbit.
Medial plate – forms lateral wall of the nasal cavity.
Middle nasal concha – thin plate of bone from the cribriform plate.
Superior nasal concha – above the middle nasal concha.
Superior meatus – between the superior and middle nasal conchae.
Middle meatus – below the middle nasal concha.

Ossification   *Perpendicular plate* – 1 centre.
Labyrinth – 1 centre per labyrinth.

Maxillae (Fig. 10.43)

Type   Irregular bones.

Position   Form the whole of the upper jaw.

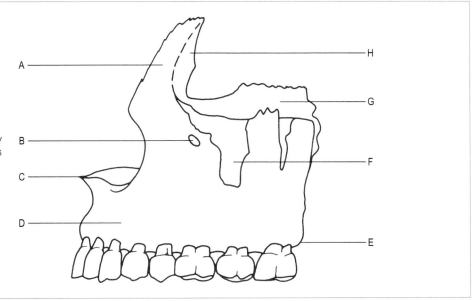

Fig. 10.43 Left maxilla (lateral aspect).
A – Frontal process
B – Infraorbital foramen
C – Anterior nasal spine
D – Canine eminence
E – Maxillary tuberosity
F – Zygomatic process
G – Orbital surface
H – Nasolacrimal groove.

Articulations

With the *opposite maxilla*, the *palatine, lacrimal, zygomatic, nasal, ethmoid* and *frontal* bones, the *inferior nasal conchae, vomer* and the *upper teeth*.

Main parts

Each bone has a body and 4 processes.

Body – pyramid-shaped and has 4 surfaces. It encloses the maxillary sinus.

Anterior surface – directed forward and laterally.

Incisive fossa – depression above the incisor teeth.

Canine fossa – depression above the canine tooth.

Canine eminence – between the 2 fossae.

Infraorbital foramen – above the canine fossa; for the infraorbital vessels and nerves.

Anterior nasal spine – a pointed process, at the junction of the 2 bodies. Infratemporal surface – convex; lies laterally.

Maxillary tuberosity – lies on the posterior aspect of the roots of the 3rd molar tooth (upper eight).

Orbital surface – forms part of the floor of the orbit.

Lacrimal notch – on the medial border of the orbital surface.

Inferior orbital fissure – anterior border is formed by the posterior border of the orbital surface.

Infraorbital canal – continuation of the infraorbital foramen.

Nasal surface – forms the wall of the nasal cavity.

Maxillary hiatus – opening on the posterior part of the nasal surface; leads to the maxillary sinus.

Conchal crest – an oblique ridge on the anterior aspect.

Zygomatic process – articulates with the zygomatic bone.

Frontal process – articulates with ethmoid, frontal, nasal and lacrimal bones; forms part of the lateral wall of the nasal cavity.

Alveolar process – forms articulation with the teeth.

Palatine process – forms part of the floor of the nasal cavity and therefore the roof of the mouth; along with the other palatine process forms three-quarters of the bony palate.

Nasal crest – at the junction of the 2 maxillae, between which is a groove for articulation with the vomer.

Maxillary sinus – see paranasal sinuses, pp. 205–210.

Ossification   3 centres.

Mandible (Figs 10.44 and 10.45)

Type   Irregular bone.

Position   Forms the lower jaw.

Articulations   *The head of mandible* with the mandibular fossa of the temporal bone to form the temporomandibular joint.
With the lower teeth.

Main parts   The bone is formed by a body and 2 rami.

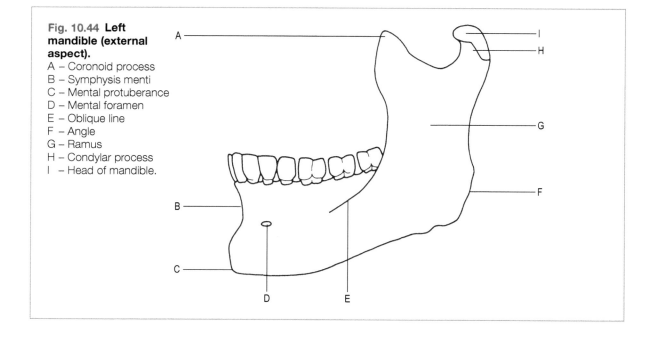

Fig. 10.44 Left mandible (external aspect).
A – Coronoid process
B – Symphysis menti
C – Mental protuberance
D – Mental foramen
E – Oblique line
F – Angle
G – Ramus
H – Condylar process
I – Head of mandible.

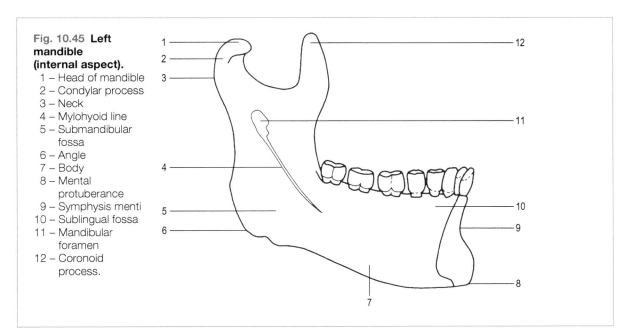

Fig. 10.45 Left mandible (internal aspect).
1 – Head of mandible
2 – Condylar process
3 – Neck
4 – Mylohyoid line
5 – Submandibular fossa
6 – Angle
7 – Body
8 – Mental protuberance
9 – Symphysis menti
10 – Sublingual fossa
11 – Mandibular foramen
12 – Coronoid process.

Body
The horseshoe-shaped aspect of the bone.

External surface – convex and subcutaneous.

Symphysis menti – in the midline where the 2 halves of the body join.

Mental protuberance – base of the symphysis menti.

Mental foramen – below the 2nd premolar tooth (lower four); carries the mental nerve and vessels.

Oblique line – continuation of the anterior border of the ramus.

Internal surface – concave.

Mylohyoid line – oblique ridge for attachment of the muscles of the pharynx.

Submandibular fossa – lies below the mylohyoid line, for the submandibular salivary glands and lymph nodes.

Sublingual fossa – above the mylohyoid line, for the sublingual salivary glands.

Ramus
Flat plate of bone at right angles to the body.

Mandibular foramen – on the medial aspect, and is the opening of the mandibular canal.

Mandibular canal – carries the mental nerve and vessel. Divides into 2 canals:

- *mental canal* – opens at the mental foramen
- *incisive canal* – opens at the incisor teeth.

Angle of the mandible – junction of the body and the ramus.

Coronoid process – triangular; forms the anterior aspect of the superior border of the ramus.

Condylar process – posterior aspect of the superior border of the ramus.

Head of mandible – expanded part of the condylar process; articulates with the mandibular fossa of the temporal bone.

Neck – narrow portion below the head.

Ossification

Primary centres

Body – 2 centres.

Secondary centres

Ramus – 4 centres.

Radiographic appearances of the mandible (Fig. 10.46)

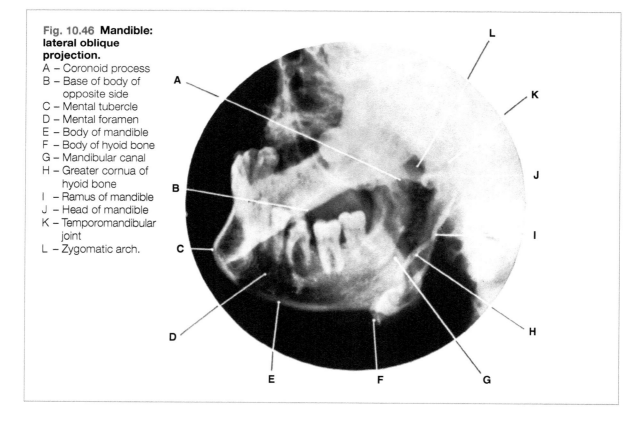

Fig. 10.46 Mandible: lateral oblique projection.
A – Coronoid process
B – Base of body of opposite side
C – Mental tubercle
D – Mental foramen
E – Body of mandible
F – Body of hyoid bone
G – Mandibular canal
H – Greater cornua of hyoid bone
I – Ramus of mandible
J – Head of mandible
K – Temporomandibular joint
L – Zygomatic arch.

Teeth

Position	Lie in the alveolar ridges of the maxillae and mandible.
Articulations	Fibrous gomphose joints between the *teeth* and *alveoli.*
Main parts (Fig. 10.47)	*Crown* – area above the gum.
	Root – embedded in the alveoli (sockets) in the mandible and maxillae.
	Neck – constriction between the root and the crown.
	Pulp cavity – central canal(s) of the tooth.
Structure	*Enamel* – dense, white, avascular structure covering the crown; approximately 1.5mm thick, mainly formed by calcium phosphate.
	Dentine – hard, yellow or white, avascular structure, similar to bone. Small canals from the dentine open into the pulp cavity.
	Dental pulp – connective tissue with blood vessels, nerves and lymphatic vessels; found in the pulp cavity.
	Apical foramen – at the apex of the root. For the passage of blood vessels and nerves.
	Cement – layer of bone-like tissue, continuous with the enamel and covering the root.

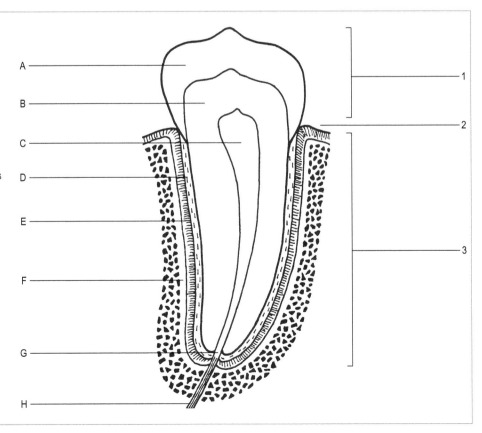

Fig. 10.47 Lower premolar tooth (coronal section).
A – Enamel
B – Dentine
C – Pulp cavity
D – Cement
E – Periodontal membrane
F – Lamina dura
G – Apical foramen
H – Nerve and vessels
1 – Crown
2 – Neck
3 – Root.

Periodontal membrane – attaches the cement to the root socket.

Lamina dura – a compact layer of bone forming the cortex of the socket in which the tooth lies.

Types of teeth

Incisors
Sharp, chisel-shaped crown, single root.
Function – biting and cutting food.

Canines
Blunt, pointed crown, single root.
Function – grasping and tearing food.

Premolars
2 cusps: 1 labial and 1 lingual. Usually a single, grooved root but upper four often have 2 roots.
Function – grinding and chewing food.

Molars
Largest teeth; occlusal surface cuboidal with 3 or 4 cusps. The upper molars have 3 roots; the lower have 2 roots.
Function – grinding and chewing food.

Dentition

Deciduous teeth
Children have a full dentition of 20 teeth: 2 incisors, 1 canine and 2 molars in each quadrant of the mouth.

Permanent teeth (Fig. 10.48)
Adults have a full dentition of 32 teeth: 2 incisors, 1 canine, 2 premolars and 3 molars in each quadrant.

Dental formulae

In order to identify the different teeth in the mouth, a formula is used. Numbers are used to identify permanent teeth:

$$\text{R} \ \frac{87654321 \ \vert \ 12345678}{87654321 \ \vert \ 12345678} \ \text{L}$$

Letters are used to identify deciduous teeth:

$$\text{R} \ \frac{\text{edcba} \ \vert \ \text{abcde}}{\text{edcba} \ \vert \ \text{abcde}} \ \text{L}$$

INSIGHT

To identify an individual tooth, part of the grid and the tooth are given, e.g.

Upper right 1 would be

$$1 \ \rceil$$

Lower left 4 would be

$$\lceil \ 4$$

Fig. 10.48 Permanent teeth – right upper and lower quadrants.
1 2 – Incisors
3 – Canine
4 5 – Premolars
6 7 8 – Molars.

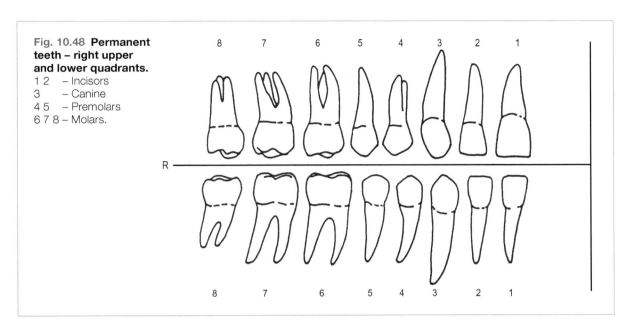

Radiographic appearances of the teeth (Figs 10.49 and 10.50)

Fig. 10.49 Teeth: intraoral projection $\overline{8765}$.
(From Bryan 1996.)
A – Erupting sac
B – Apex of root
C – Lamina dura
D – Periodontal membrane
E – Pulp cavity
F – Enamel of crown
G – Radio-opaque filling.

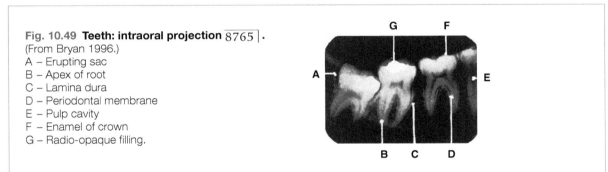

Pathology

Edentulous – without teeth.

Gingivitis – inflammation of the gums caused by a build-up of dental plaque.

Dental caries – decay often caused by poor diet or poor dental hygiene.

Periodontal disease – in the early stages presents as gingivitis; in later stages affects the structure and support of the teeth causing loosening.

Abscess – a cavity containing pus; the most common site is on the apex of the root of the tooth.

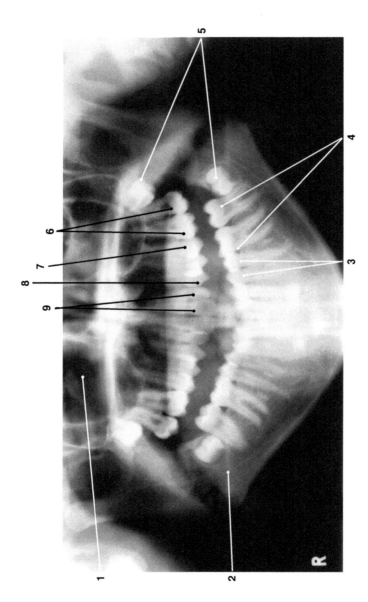

Fig. 10.50 Teeth: orthopantomograph.
1 – Maxillary antrum
2 – Mandibular canal
3 – Pre-molars
4 – Molars
5 – Unerupted 3rd molars (bilateral)
6 – Molars
7 – Premolar
8 – Canine
9 – Incisors.

Inferior nasal conchae

Type	Irregular bones.
Position	Lie on the lateral walls of the nasal cavity.
Articulations	With the *maxillae, ethmoid, palatine* and *lacrimal* bones.
Main parts	Each bone has 2 surfaces, 2 borders and 2 ends.

Medial surface – convex.

Lateral surface – forms part of the inferior meatus of the nasal cavity.

Superior border – the middle of which presents 3 processes:

- *lacrimal process* – forms part of the nasolacrimal canal
- *ethmoidal process* – articulates with the ethmoid bone
- *maxillary process* – forms part of the medial wall of the maxillary sinus.

Inferior border – non-articular.

Ends of the bone – pointed.

Ossification	1 primary centre.

Lacrimal bones

Type	Irregular bone.
Position	Lie on the medial wall of the orbits.
Articulation	With the *maxillae, ethmoid* and *frontal* bones and the *inferior nasal conchae*.
Main parts	The bones have 2 surfaces and 4 borders each.

Lateral or orbital surface – is divided by a vertical crest.

Posterior lacrimal crest – divides the lateral surface.

Fossa for the lacrimal sac – formed where the crest articulates with the maxilla; forms part of the canal for the nasolacrimal duct.

Lacrimal hamulus – a hook at the end of the crest.

Medial or nasal surface – forms the middle meatus of the nose and articulates with the ethmoid bone.

Anterior border – articulates with the maxilla.

Posterior border – articulates with the ethmoid bone.

Superior border – articulates with the frontal bone.

Inferior border – articulates with the maxilla.

Ossification	1 primary centre.

Nasal bones

Type	Flat bones.
Position	Form the bridge of the nose.
Articulations	With the *frontal* bone, *maxilla,* the *ethmoid* bone and the other *nasal* bone; is continuous with the cartilage of the nasal septum.
Main parts	The bone has 2 surfaces and 4 borders.
	External surface – concavoconvex.
	Internal surface – groove for anterior ethmoid nerve.
	Superior border – articulates with the frontal bone at the nasion.
	Inferior border – articulates with the cartilage of the nasal septum.
	Lateral border – articulates with the maxilla.
	Medial border – articulates with the ethmoid, frontal and other nasal bone.
Ossification	1 primary centre.

Vomer

Type	Flat bone.
Position	Forms the postero-inferior aspect of the bony nasal septum.
Articulations	With the *maxillae, sphenoid, ethmoid,* and *palatine* bones and the cartilage of the nasal septum.
Main parts	The bone has 2 surfaces and 4 borders.
	Superior surface – has small grooves for blood vessels and nerves.
	Inferior surface – has small grooves for blood vessels and nerves.
	Superior border – thick, and has a deep furrow.
	Alae – projections from the superior border; articulate with the sphenoid and palatine bones.
	Inferior border – articulates with the nasal crest of the maxillae and palatine bones.
	Anterior border – articulates with ethmoid and nasal septum (cartilaginous part).
	Posterior border – separates the posterior nasal apertures.
Ossification	2 primary centres.

Palatine bones

Type	Irregular bones.
Position	They lie in the posterior part of the nasal and oral cavities.

Articulations	With the *maxillae, vomer, inferior nasal conchae, sphenoid* and *ethmoid* bones and the other *palatine* bone.
Main parts	The bones are L-shaped and each has a horizontal and a vertical plate.

Horizontal plate

Has 2 surfaces and 4 borders.

Nasal surface – forms part of the floor of the nasal cavity.

Palatine surface – forms the posterior part of the bony palate.

Posterior border – has a pointed medial end, which forms the posterior nasal spine.

Posterior nasal spine – forms attachment for the uvula.

Anterior border – articulates with the maxilla.

Lateral border – unites the horizontal and perpendicular plates.

Medial border – articulates with the other palatine bone, forming the posterior part of the nasal crest.

Perpendicular plate

Has 2 surfaces and 4 borders.

Nasal surface – forms part of the inferior meatus of the nasal cavity and has 2 crests.

Conchal crest – articulates with the inferior nasal concha.

Ethmoidal crest – articulates with the middle nasal concha.

Middle meatus – part of this lies between the 2 crests.

Maxillary surface – articulates with the maxilla and (along with the anterior border of the perpendicular plate) forms part of the medial wall of the maxillary sinus.

Posterior border – articulates with the sphenoid bone.

Superior border – has 2 large processes.

- *orbital process* – articulates with the maxilla and ethmoid; forms part of the floor of the orbit and the inferior orbital fissure.
- *sphenoidal process* – articulates with the sphenoid bone; forms part of the roof and lateral wall of the nasal cavity.

Sphenopalatine notch – lies between the 2 processes.

Pyramidal process – lies at the junction of the horizontal and perpendicular plates; articulates with the maxilla and sphenoid bone.

Ossification	*Perpendicular plate* – 1 primary centre.

Zygomatic bones

Type	Irregular bones.
Position	Forms the bony cheek and part of the lateral walls and the floor of the orbit.

Articulations	With the *maxilla, temporal, frontal* and *sphenoid* bones.
Main parts	Each bone has 3 surfaces, 5 borders and 2 processes.

Lateral surface – convex; projects laterally and forwards.

Temporal surface – concave; projects medially and backwards.

Orbital surface – concave; forms part of the floor and lateral wall of the orbit.

Orbital border – concave; forms the inferior and lateral aspects of the orbital margin.

Maxillary border – articulates with the maxilla.

Temporal border – convex; articulates with the frontal bone forming part of the lateral wall of the orbit.

Postero-inferior border – forms attachment for the masseter muscle.

Postero-medial border – articulates with maxilla and the sphenoid bone forming the zygomaticofrontal suture.

Frontal process – articulates with the frontal and sphenoid bone.

Temporal process – articulates with the temporal bone and forms part of the zygomatic arch.

Ossification	1 primary centre.

Hyoid bone

Type	Irregular bone.
Position	Lies in the front of the neck, above the thyroid cartilage of the larynx at the root of the tongue.
Articulations	The bone is attached to the *temporal bone* by the stylohyoid ligament.
Main parts	*Body* – convex.

Greater cornua – project back laterally from the body.

Lesser cornua – project upwards at the junction between the body and the greater cornua.

The bone gives attachment for muscles of the mouth, tongue and middle constrictor muscle of the pharynx.

Ossification	Primary centres

Body – 2 centres.

Greater cornua – 2 centres.

Lesser cornua – 2 centres.

Radiographic appearances of the facial bones (Figs 10.51, 10.52 and 10.53)

Fig. 10.51 Facial bones: occipitomental projection.
(From Bryan 1996.)
A – Nasal bones
B – Frontozygomatic suture
C – Zygomatic bone
D – Maxillary sinus
E – Coronoid process of mandible
F – Ramus of mandible
G – Angle of mandible
H – Petrous part of temporal bone
I – Mastoid air cells
J – Head of mandible
K – Zygomatic arch
L – Infraorbital foramen
M – Lesser wing of sphenoid
N – Nasal septum
O – Supraorbital margin
P – Frontal sinus.

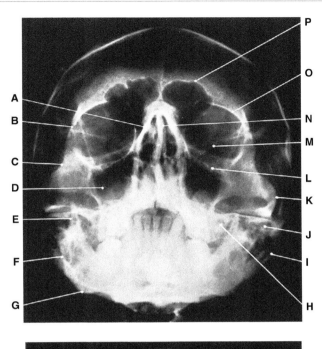

Fig. 10.52 Facial bones: 30° occipitomental projection.
(From Bryan 1996.)
1 – Zygomatic arch
2 – Coronoid process
3 – Maxilla
4 – Infraorbital margin.

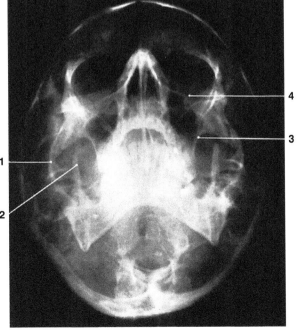

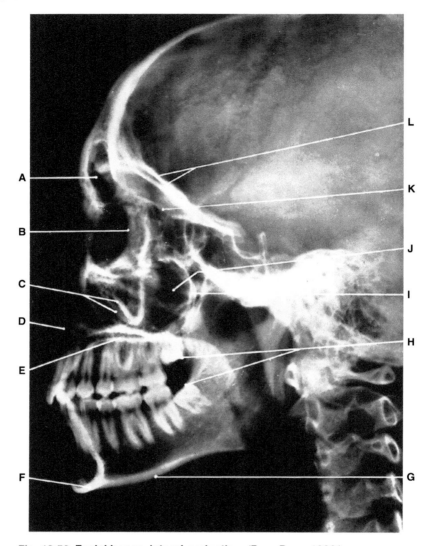

Fig. 10.53 Facial bones: lateral projection. (From Bryan 1996.)

A – Frontal sinuses
B – Lateral margin or orbit
C – Zygomatic processes of maxillae
D – Anterior nasal spine
E – Hard palate
F – Mental tubercle
G – Base of mandible
H – Unerupted third molars
I – Posterior surface of maxilla
J – Maxillary sinuses
K – Cribriform plate of ethmoid bone
L – Orbital plates of frontal bone.

TEMPOROMANDIBULAR JOINT (Fig. 10.54)

Type	Synovial condylar joint.
Bony articular surfaces	Articular tubercle and the anterior aspect of the mandibular fossa of the temporal bone above, with the condyle of the mandible below. The articular surfaces are covered with white fibrocartilage.
Fibrous capsule	Surrounds the joint; it is attached to the articular tubercle, and the circumference of the mandibular fossa and the neck of mandible. The capsule is loose above and tight below.
Synovial membrane	Lines the fibrous capsule. The membrane secretes synovial fluid, which lubricates the joint.
Supporting ligaments	*Lateral (temporomandibular) ligament* – from the zygoma to the neck of the mandible. *Sphenomandibular ligament* – from the spine of the sphenoid to the lingula of the mandibular foramen. *Stylomandibular ligament* – from the styloid process to the angle and ramus of the mandible.
Intracapsular structure	*Articular disc* – fibrous tissue, divides the joint cavity horizontally into 2 sections and is fused with the capsule.
Movements	*Depression* by the lateral pterygoid muscle.

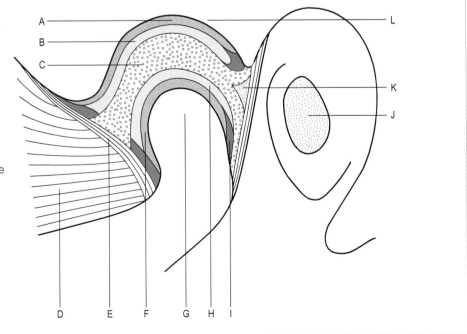

Fig. 10.54 Left temporomandibular joint (sagittal section)
A – Fibrocartilage
B – Synovial fluid
C – Articular disc
D – Lateral pterygoid ligament
E – Fibrous capsule
F – Fibrocartilage
G – Head of mandible
H – Synovial fluid
I – Synovial membrane
J – External acoustic meatus
K – Venous plexus
L – Mandibular fossa

Elevation by the temporalis, masseter and medial pterygoid muscles.
Protrusion by the lateral and medial pterygoid muscles.
Retraction by the temporalis muscle.
Lateral movement by the medial and lateral pterygoid muscles.

Blood supply   Superficial temporal and maxillary arteries.

Nerve supply   Branches of the mandibular nerve.

Radiographic appearances of the temporomandibular joint (Figs 10.55, 10.56, 10.57 and 10.58)

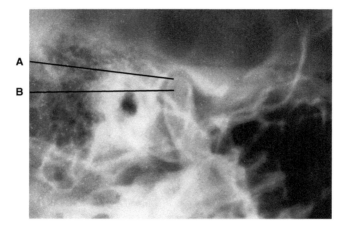

Fig. 10.55 Temporomandibular joint: lateral oblique projection with mouth closed. (From Bryan 1996.)
A – Mandibular fossa of temporal bone
B – Head of mandible.

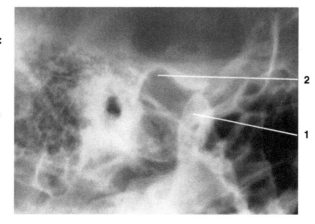

Fig. 10.56 Temporomandibular joint: lateral oblique projection with mouth open.
(From Bryan 1996.)
1 – Head of mandible
2 – Mandibular fossa of temporal bone.

Fig. 10.57 **Temporo-mandibular joint mouth closed. MR scan.** (From Resnick Kransdorf, 2005.)

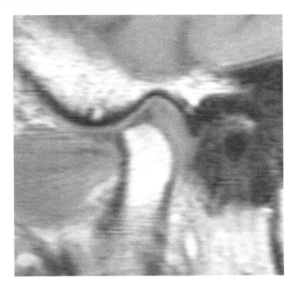

Fig. 10.58 **Temporo-mandibular joint mouth open. MR scan.** (From Resnick Kransdorf, 2005.)

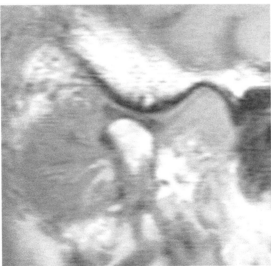

Fractures

Cranium

Either a hairline fracture or a depressed fracture.

Cause – blow to the head; may result in a haematoma (subdural or extradural).

Example of treatment – bed rest with regular neurological checks; depressed fractures may require elevating.

Zygomatic arch	Cause – blow to the cheek. Example of treatment – depressed fracture is raised during open surgery as the fracture is then stable; no immobilisation is required.
Mandible	(Fig. 10.59)

Due to the rigidity of the temporomandibular joints, a fracture of the mandible will always result in a second fracture of the mandible or a fracture dislocation of the temporomandibular joint on the opposite side. Think of a polo mint – it is impossible to break it in one place.

Fig. 10.59 Fractured mandible. (From Sutton 1987.)

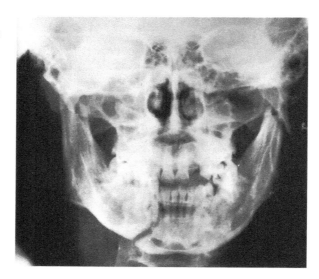

Always 2 fracture lines or a fracture dislocation. Most common sites are the lower premolar region (lower four region) and the opposite condylar neck, or both condylar necks.

Cause – oblique blow to the jaw.

Example of treatment – the maxilla and the mandible may be wired together.

Maxilla	The most common region, the lower orbital rim, tends to cause bleeding into the maxillary sinus, which can be demonstrated radiographically using a horizontal beam technique (blood in the sinus shows as an area of increased density). *Cause* – blow to the orbit. *Example of treatment* – reduction under general anaesthetic. Immobilisation by either wiring to the mandible or wire from the teeth to a metal rod attached to a head plaster.

Pathology

Hydrocephalus

Malformation of the medulla and 4th ventricle with blockage of the opening resulting in accumulation of cerebrospinal fluid and therefore enlarged ventricles. If not controlled the skull vault becomes enlarged.

Example of treatment – either a drain is inserted between one or both of the ventricles and the cisterna magna, or a unidirectional valve is inserted between the ventricles and the vena cava or the right atrium.

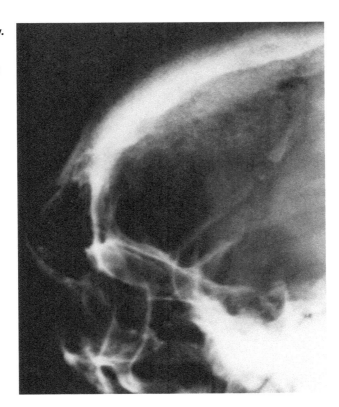

Fig. 10.60 Acromegaly. Note the thickened cranium, prominent sinuses and supraorbital ridges and enlarged pituitary fossa. (From Resnick Kransdorf, 2005.)

Pituitary fossa
(Fig. 10.60)

Enlargement may indicate an adenoma and therefore the cause of acromegaly, gigantism or Cushing's disease.

Diminished size may indicate atrophy of the pituitary gland and therefore a cause of amenorrhea.

Facial bones

Infection of the maxillary sinus may result in mucosal thickening or fluid in the cavity. This can be demonstrated with an occipitomental radiograph.

Glossary

A– Absence of.

Abduction To move away from the midline.

Abscess A cavity containing pus.

Achondroplasia Lack of bone growth due to a gene defect.

Acromegaly Excessive secretion of the growth hormone causing thickening of the bones of the skull, mandible, hands and feet.

Adactyly Absence of fingers.

Adduction To move towards the midline.

Amelia Absence of fingers.

Amphiarthroses Cartilaginous joints.

Ankylosing spondylitis Inflammatory disorder of the joints of the spinal column.

Anterior Nearer the front of the body.

Atlas 1st cervical vertebra.

Auricular Ear-shaped.

Axis A line of the body, 2nd cervical vertebra.

Bi– Two or twice.

Biaxial Movement round two lines of the body.

Bipartite Split into two.

Brachy– Short.

Brachydactyly Short phalanges.

Brachymesophalangy Short middle phalanges.

Buccal Near the cheek.

CDH Congenital dislocation of the hip.

Caisson disease Bone necrosis affecting people who experience high atmospheric pressure.

Canal Bony tunnel.

Canaliculi Channels carrying nutrient fluid in compact bone.

Caries Decay, usually of teeth.

Carrying angle Medial angle between the long axis of the humerus and the ulna.

Cervical rib An extra rib, usually attached to the 7th cervical vertebra.

Chondro– Relating to cartilage.

Chondroma A tumour of mature cartilage.

Chondrosarcoma A primary tumour of cartilage, usually affecting the long bones.

Circumduction Combination of movements to make a circle.

Circumferential lamellae Rings of bone round the circumference of compact bone.

Club foot Twisting of the foot from the normal shape.

Colles' fracture Fracture of the lower end of radius with posterior and lateral displacement of the distal fragment.

Comminuted Containing a number of pieces of bone.

Compression Crushed.

Condyle Smooth, rounded area, often articular.

Congenital talipes equino-varies Congenital club foot.

Contrecoup An injury caused by a blow to the opposite side of an area e.g. pelvis or skull.

Cortex Outer layer (of bone).

Costal Associated with the ribs.

Coxa vara Deformity of the femur when the angle between the neck and the shaft is reduced resulting in the shortening of the leg.

Crest A sharp ridge.

CT Computed tomography, demonstrates anatomical abnormality.

Cusp Rounded projection.

Dactyly Phalanges.

Demi– Half.

Diarthroses Synovial joints.

Dislocation Complete displacement of two bones in a joint.

Distal The outer end or farthest away towards the back of the mouth.

Dorsal Nearer the back of the body.

Dys– Painful, abnormal.

Dysplasia Abnormal growth.

Dystrophy Abnormal activity of cells due to poor nutrition.

Edentulous Without teeth.

Emphysema, surgical Air in the tissues.

Epi– Above.

Epicondyle An elevation above a condyle.

Ewing's sarcoma Malignant tumour thought to be of the reticuloendothelial cells usually affecting long bones or the pelvis.

Extension Straightening of a joint.

External Outside.

External rotation Turn outwards.

Facet Smooth area, often articular.

Fibrosarcoma Malignant tumour of fibrous tissue.

Fibrous dysplasia Abnormal growth of fibrous tissue which may contain cysts.

Fissure Narrow slit.

^{18}FDG 18 Fluorodeoxyglucose, a radiopharmaceutical used in PET studies for tumour imaging.

Flexion Bending a joint.

Fluorosis Staining of the teeth as a result of taking excess fluoride.

^{18}F-NaF Sodium fluoride used in bone scans to demonstrate bone metastasis.

Foramen Hole.

Fossa Wide depression.

Galeazzi's fracture Fracture of the lower third of radius with dislocation of the head of ulna.

Gigantism Excessive growth due to abnormal secretion of the growth hormone.

Gingivitis Inflammation of gums.

Gliding Sliding.

Gout A metabolic disorder resulting in uric acid in a joint space, inflammation and pain.

Greenstick fracture An incomplete break.

Groove Uncovered passage.

Hamulus Hook-like projection.

Haversian canal A channel in compact bone containing blood, lymphatic vessels and nerves.

Haversian systems The microscopic structure of compact bone.

Hallux valgus Lateral deviation of great toe from first metatarsal.

Haemophilia Excessive bleeding which can result in bleeding into joint cavities.

Haemothorax Blood in the pleural cavity.

Hemi– Half, affecting one side.

Hemimelia Absence of part of the hand.

Hemivertebra Half a vertebra.

Hyper– More, high.

Hyperparathyroidism Excess of parathormone which can result in a loss of calcium from bones.

Hyperphalangism More phalanges.

Hypo Less, low.

Impacted One item pushed into another.

Inferior Below.

Infra– Below.

Innominate bone Hip bone.

Inter– Between.

Internal Inside.

Internal rotation Turn inwards.

Interstitial lamella The spaces between the haversian systems in compact bone.

Intra– Within.

Ischaemia Insufficient blood supply.

Kyphosis Excessive spinal curvature.

Labial Next to the lips.

Lacunae Space between the lamellae of compact bone.

Lamellae Microscopic rings of bone, round a haversian canal.

Lamina Thin plate.

Lateral Away from the midline of the body.

Leukaemia Excess of white blood cells in the bone marrow.

Line Long, narrow ridge.

Lingual Next to the tongue.

Lordosis Excessive secondary curvature of the spine.

Lumbago Pain in the region of the lumbar spine.

Macro– Large.

Macrodactyly Enlargement of a digit.

Meatus Narrow passage.

Medial Nearer the midline of the body.

Melia Limb.

Mesial Towards the front or the midline.

Monteggia's fracture Fracture of the upper third of ulna with dislocation of the head of radius.

99mTc-MDP Technetium methylene diphosphonate, a radiopharmaceutical administered for SPECT scintigraphy.

Multiaxial Movement round more than 2 lines of the body.

Multipartite Split into pieces.

Myelomatosis Tumour of the bone marrow.

NAI Non-accidental injury.

Necrosis 'Bone death' resulting from the loss of blood supply to the area.

Notch Large groove.

Occlusal Biting edge.

Oligodactyly Absence of fingers.

Osgood–Schlatter's disease Condition affecting the tibial tuberosity.

Ossification The formation of bone from connective tissue.

Osteo– Bone.

Osteoblastoma Tumour of the osteoblasts.

Osteoblasts Bone cells which build bone.

Osteoclasts Bone cells which destroy or shape bone.

Osteochondritis Bone necrosis causing fragmentation of bone.

Osteochondroma Tumour of cartilaginous cells.

Osteoclastoma Tumour of the osteoclasts.

Osteocytes Mature bone cells.

Osteoma Benign bone tumour, involving the osteoblast cells.

Osteomalacia Decrease of bone calcification due to lack of vitamin D.

Osteomyelitis Bone infection, causing bone destruction, treated with antibiotics.

Osteonecrosis Loss of blood supply to bone.

Osteopetrosis Deficiency of osteoclasts causing an increase in bone density.

Osteoporosis Loss of bone matrix resulting in brittle bones and therefore fractures.

Osteosarcoma A malignant tumour of bone, can rapidly spread to the lungs.

Osteosclerosis See osteopetrosis.

Paget's disease Balance between bone building and bone destruction is disturbed, affected bones are prone to fracture.

Palatal Next to the palate.

Periodontal Round a tooth.

Periosteum A membrane which surrounds all bone, except the articular surfaces.

Perthes' disease Inflammation of the epiphysis of the femoral head.

Pes planus Flat feet.

PET Positron Emission Tomography, demonstrates functional abnormality.

PET/CT Combining (or fusing) PET and CT images to demonstrate the accurate anatomical location of the functional abnormality.

PFFD Proximal femoral focal deficiency (congenitally short femur).

Phocomelia Absence of the proximal part of a limb.

Pneumothorax Air in the pleural cavity.

Poly– Increase in, more.

Polydactyly Increase in the number of digits.

Posterior Nearer the back of the body.

Pott's fracture Fracture dislocation of the ankle.

Process Localised projection.

Proximal Towards the trunk.

Radiopharmaceutical A radioactive compound used in scintigraphy.

Rheumatoid arthritis Inflammatory joint disease which affects many joints.

Scheuermann's disease Adolescent kyphosis.

Sciatica Pain along the sciatic nerve, usually round the buttock or thigh.

Scintigraphy Radionuclide imaging

Sesamoid bones Bones which develop in tendons.

Skeletal scintigraphy Radionuclide Imaging or Isotope Bone Scan.

Smith's fracture Fracture of the distal end of the radius with anterior displacement of the distal fragment.

SPECT Single Photon Emission Computed Tomography, demonstrates functional abnormality.

SPECT/CT Combining (or fusing) SPECT and CT images to demonstrate the accurate anatomical location of the functional abnormality.

Spina bifida Incomplete fusion of the neural arches.

Spine Long process.

Spondyl A vertebra.

Spondylolisthesis Moving forward of one vertebra on another, usually 5th lumbar vertebra on the 1st sacral vertebra.

Squamous Thin, flat, scale-like.

Still's disease Juvenile rheumatoid arthritis.

Sub– Below or nearly.

Subluxation Partial dislocation.

Sulcus Groove or furrow.

Supra– Above.

Superior Above.

Symphalangism Fusion of the phalanges.

Synarthroses Fibrous joints.

Syndactyly Fusion of adjacent digits.

Synostosis Fusion of adjacent bones.

Trochanter Large, rounded, elevation.

Trochlea Pulley-shaped surface.

Tubercle Small, rounded, elevation.

Tuberosity Large, rounded, elevation.

Uniaxial Movement round one line of the body.

Ventral Nearer the front of the body.

Volkmann's canals Canals joining haversian canals.

Index

Note: Page numbers followed by *b* indicates boxes, *f* indicates figures and *t* indicates tables.

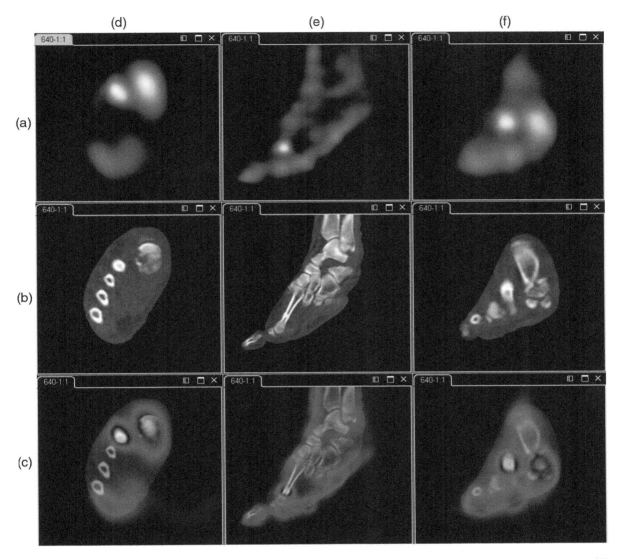

(d)   (e)   (f)

Plate 1 **Osteomyelitis of 1st and 2nd distal metatarsals.** Gallium-67 (a) SPECT images (b) corresponding CT images and (c) fused SPECT/CT images, (d) axial, (e) sagittal and (f) coronal views. (Courtesy of Philips Healthcare.)

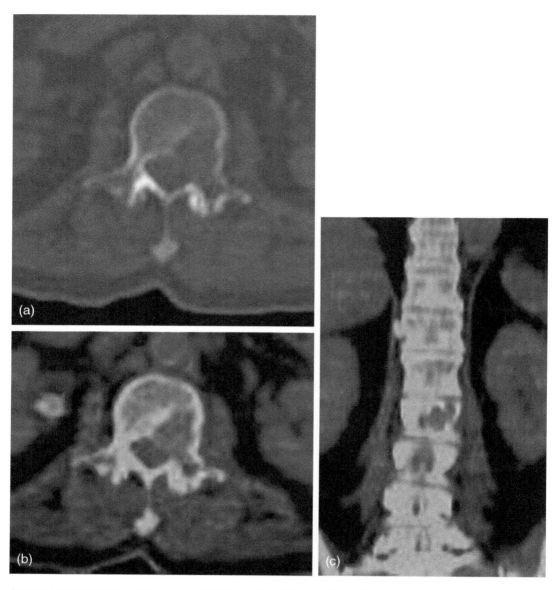

Plate 2 Vertebral Body Metastasis. PET/CT. (a) Axial CT (b) axial and (c) coronal fused PET/CT. (Courtesy of Vidhiya Vinayakamoorthy. Images © InHealth 2010.)

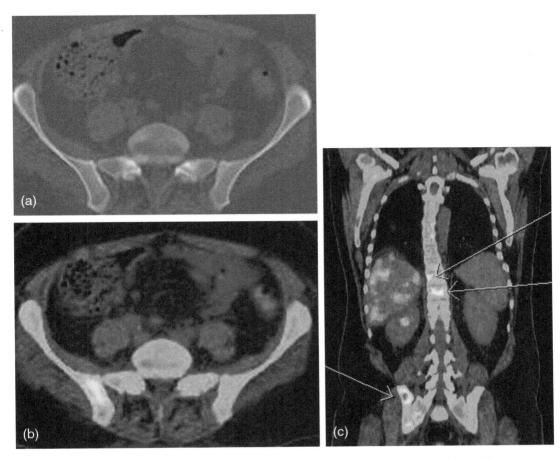

Plate 3 Lymphoma with widespread bony deposits. PET/CT. (a) Axial CT and fused (b) axial and (c) coronal PET/CT. (Courtesy of Vidhiya Vinayakamoorthy. Images © Inhealth 2010.)

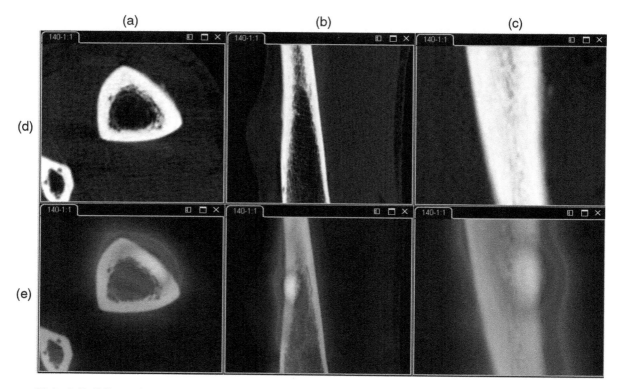

Plate 4 Soft tissue tumour extension into bone. SPECT/CT. 99mTc-MDP CT images, (a) axial (b) sagittal and (c) coronal views, corresponding (d) CT and (e) fused SPECT/CT images. (Courtesy of Philips Healthcare.)

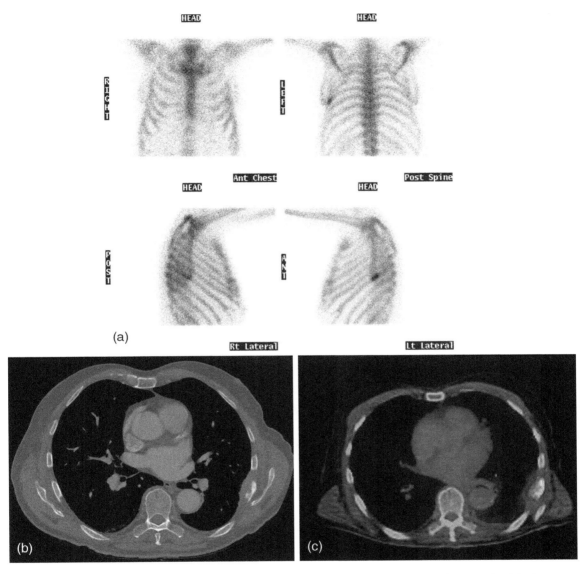

Plate 5 Direct rib invasion by pleural mesothelioma. (a) Skeletal scintigraphy shows increased uptake in rib. (b) ^{18}F NaF PET/CT- showing soft tissue mass destroying rib. (c) Fused PET/CT images. (Courtesy of Vidhiya Vinayakamoorthy. Images © InHealth 2010.)

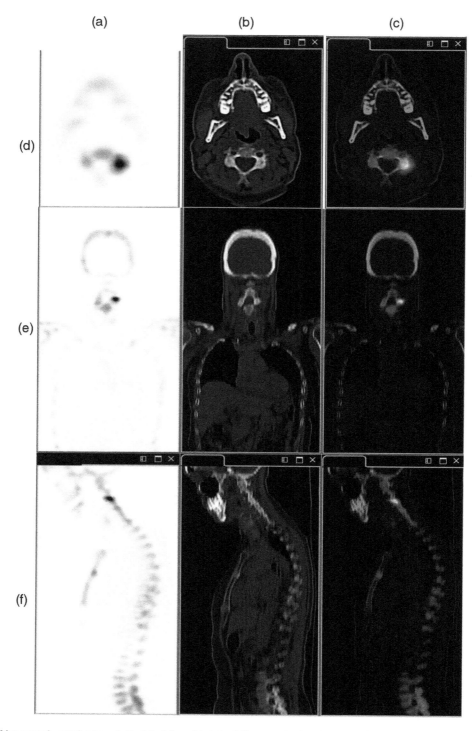

Plate 6 Abnormal uptake in a left sided facet joint of the cervical spine. PET/CT. (a) ^{18}F NaF PET images, (b) CT images and (c) fused PET/CT images (d) axial, (e) coronal and (f) sagittal views. (Courtesy of Philips Healthcare.)

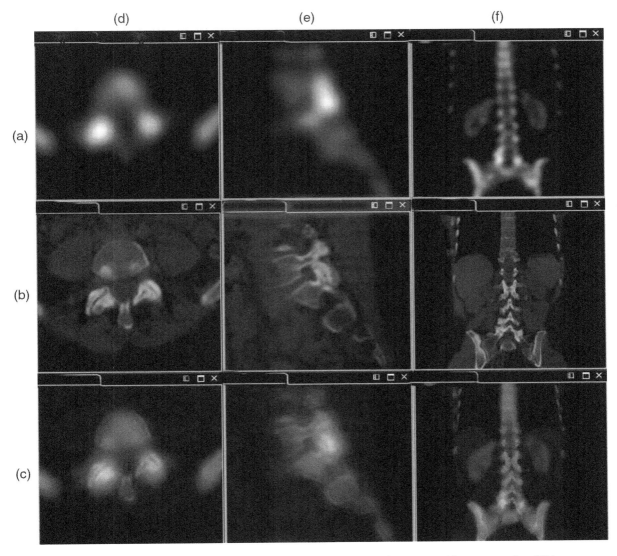

(d)   (e)   (f)

(a)

(b)

(c)

Plate 7 **Facet disease of the spine SPECT/CT.** 99mTcMDP (a) SPECT Images, (b) corresponding CT images and (c) fused SPECT/CT images. (d) axial, (e) sagittal and (f) coronal views. (Courtesy of Philips Healthcare.)

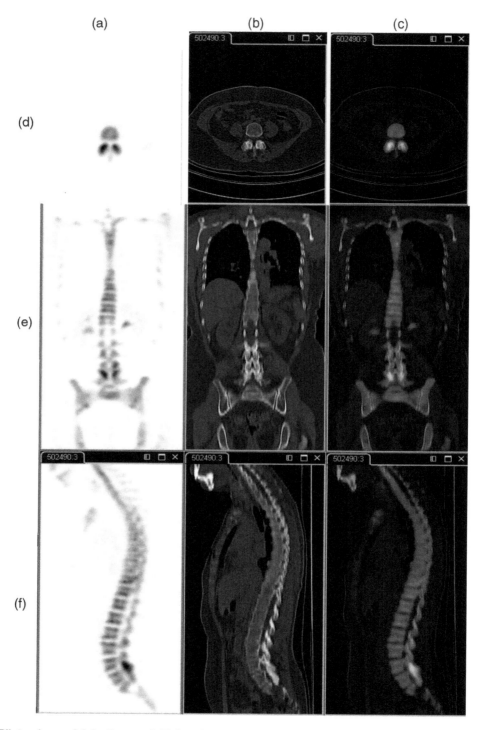

Plate 8 Bilateral spondylolystheses at 4th Lumbar vertebra PET/CT. (a) 99m Tc-MDP CT images, (b) CT images and (c) fused PET/CT images, (d) axial, (e) coronal and (f) sagittal. (Courtesy of Philips Healthcare.)